# Since The Days Of
# The Romans

# SINCE THE DAYS OF
# THE ROMANS

*My journey of
discovering a life with horses*

# GEOFF TUCKER D.V.M.

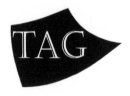

TAG Publishing, LLC
2030 S. Milam
Amarillo, TX 79109
www.TAGPublishers.com
Office (806) 373-0114
Fax (806) 373-4004
info@TAGPublishers.com

ISBN: 978-1-934606-53-7

First Edition

Copyright © 2014 Geoff Tucker

Quantity discounts are available on bulk orders.
Contact info@TAGPublishers.com for more information.

# CONTENTS

# SINCE THE DAYS OF THE ROMANS

I was looking forward to a pleasant, routine call as I turned up the long driveway leading to a farm located in the hills at the southern end of my practice. My client had scheduled Coggins tests, vaccinations and teeth floating for her two horses. I could see that no one was in the barn, so I walked to the house.

In outside appearance, the two-story, white clapboard colonial looked typical for the area. I entered the garage and knocked on the house door calling out, "Dr. Tucker -- anyone home?"

A distant voice replied, "Come on into the kitchen, Doc."

I was hit with warm moist air and my nostrils filled with chlorine as I passed through the first room of the house with its hidden pool. It made me think that this wealthy woman believed in healthy living in the cold, upstate New

York area. But the hidden pool, like an oasis inside the old farmhouse, wasn't what was unusual about my "routine" call that day.

The woman, a new client for me, was sitting at her kitchen table. Clear morning light poured through the large window over the sink passing through hand made white linen curtains spotted with colorful shapes of vegetables. Tucked into the corner of the room, the table had the hallmark of being the social center of the house. The smell of coffee added warmth.

A man was seated and he was quickly introduced to me as her guest. His appearance was itself unusual because he was not dressed in a way that was typical for the area. Men usually wore work boots and functional clothing on the farms I visit. While the woman wore clothes for barn chores, this man wore pressed slacks, a long sleeved Oxford shirt with button down collar, and a dark-brown, Cashmere wool sweater vest. His head was topped with the type of cap that called up images of Sherlock Holmes, and he wore black, leather loafers with tassels that were definitely not suited for farm work.

He seemed proper, relaxed and professional. I knew that her guest was not a horseman but was surprised with her candid introduction when she said, "He's my psychotherapist."

Well, I thought to myself, I know plenty of horse people who might benefit from hiring a psychotherapist including myself. Noting their apparent comfort with each other, I also wondered to myself exactly what kind of therapy he was providing in addition to his regular services.

I was asked permission for him to come to the barn to see what kind of work I did, and I happily agreed thinking I may glean therapeutic benefit for myself during the visit. We all headed to the barn with the man measuring his steps in an attempt to keep his loafers clean. I never expected him to be the man to confirm a deep-seated feeling I had been ignoring all of my life.

As I worked with the horses, I discussed basic horse care with the owner while the therapist stood by, quietly watching.

"These are two very different horses, aren't they?" he asked during a silent pause in our discussion, surprising me with his accurate assessment.

"You're very correct! These are two distinctly different horses," I answered, surprised. "Tell me, what do you see?"

"One of them seems so calm and relaxed and understanding," he said. "The other seems more aloof and inquisitive, but in a fearful sort of way."

He was exactly right. "You have nailed their personalities which surprises me since you don't have any experience with horses," I said.

He responded, "In the type of therapy I do, I read auras. I can see these horse's auras and their personalities are what I read."

I was speechless and the world stopped. It had been many years since my first job with horses. I'd learned about reading auras and incorporated it into my work with horses. It had become so much second nature that I rarely consciously thought about it. Now a non-horseman, human psychotherapist had rekindled a memory from my beginning days of working with horses in 1973.

With an effort I brought myself back to the present, where I'd just finished with the first of the horses. I turned to look at the man.

"Is there anything else you can tell me about these horses?" I asked.

"That's it," he said, and I felt a moment's disappointment before he added, "But I do read people's auras and you have a strong one."

The therapist told me that I had two strong auras, one for healing and one for teaching. I nodded, but thought privately, "Well that's a no-brainer. I'm a veterinarian, for crying out loud. Of course I'm into healing and he has just listened to me talk about horses with the owner so he knows I like to teach as I work."

"There's one more thing, Dr. Tucker," the therapist said. "But, I don't know if you want to hear it."

Well, if you want to tweak someone's curiosity, just say something like that. I couldn't just let the conversation end there. I insisted he tell me what he was feeling, even if it was something he wasn't sure I'd want to know.

The aura reader said, "This isn't the first life you've lived with horses." I felt a chill as he continued. "It's clear to me that you've been working with horses since the days of the Romans."

Unlike many equine veterinarians, I hadn't been raised around horses. However, I'd taken to them and they had taken to me with an ease that surprised me. I had always felt that I'd been around them in previous lives.

My mind flew to another memory. An old and very wise horseman who owned a farm in New York once told me, "You can live your whole life with horses, die, be born again, live your whole life again with horses, die, be born again, and so on. After many such lives, you might just start to understand them."

*Had I lived many lives with horses? Was it my destiny to live this life again with them? Why had a three-time college dropout, a kid with a reading disability, a person with no experience with horses for the first 20 years of his life, been drawn almost with Divine purpose into a life that complimented my inner being?*

*On a routine call, a man who had nothing to do with horses had given me a revelation. Maybe this wasn't my first time around with horses. Maybe I have been with them since the days of the Romans.*

# INTRODUCTION

This is a book about the adventures I have taken from just after high school through graduation from veterinary school. Those various twists and turns are interspersed with stories *in italics* of horses and their owners that I came across early in my veterinary career – every one of them true. I wrote this book because I know so many people suffer from what I have known as a life without direction and may even be tempted to give up. Leaping into unknown areas in life is upsetting and freighting. Roadblocks are annoying at best and insurmountable at worst, yet still there is hope.

I left high school unable to read well enough to have any chance at good college exam scores. I was the son of a family of Ivy League school graduates, a boy uninterested in animals, a loner with no direction, and a three-time college dropout. How could someone like me make it into the top veterinary college in the world and become successful at treating horses throughout the United States? Against all odds, I achieved what makes me happy. I had support and love along the way, which is imperative to success.

This is a story of overcoming adversity to become what life has in mind for you in spite of yourself. It is based on a life with horses but applies to every person on earth. I am not the only one to find direction and purpose in a life of chaos but my message is clear to those who may not believe this. If I can do it, then so can you.

Let's start with my thoughts about horses. A horse can kill you. It's a fact. They are large animals with minds of their own, yet horses hold an elevated position in our collective imagination. They are beautiful, graceful and have been part of human existence for thousands of years. In prior generations, those who owned horses depended on their ability to work, to transport and to make daily life easier, but they also loved their horses. Steal a man's wife and he might punch you in the mouth, but steal his horse and you'd be hung from the nearest tree!

While these days we depend much less on a horse's ability to work, horse people still love their animals not because they are pretty (though they are) or because they are easy to care for (they are not!). The love comes from a special reciprocal connection a person and a horse develop. It becomes a true friendship, one often not found between two humans.

My name is Geoff Tucker and I'm an equine veterinarian – a horse doctor. Now you may assume that I grew up on a farm or ranch or that I'd been around horses all my life and that's how I developed such a love for them. You'd be wrong.

My father was a corporate lawyer in Manhattan. That is about as far removed from a farm as any place I know. I wasn't raised with mud on my boots and straw between my teeth, but somehow, someway, I found my place in the world with horses.

When I think about it now, I wonder how in the heck I could have possibly ended-up in this line of work and loving my life. It was a long and twisting road, but one I'd travel again tomorrow if I could get the same result.

I suppose everyone at some point takes a step back and wonders how things have come together through the years to create their life. Success seems like an elusive thing for so many – so why did it happen that I became successful almost in spite of myself?

I have heard numerous definitions for success from being gifted to being the result of hard work. Though I'd certainly never call myself gifted, I do work hard. Luck is another common reason given by many for success, though I believe that the real definition of luck is when preparedness meets opportunity. I think the combination of success and happiness is much more than that though. In my case, there had to be some divine guidance involved for my very disjointed and improbable path in life to produce such results.

I never had a horse growing up. I had a dog and a cat but the cat was run over and the dog was dognapped for research. It seems that Weimaraner dogs have little hair and fat so they are useful for research and it turned out that three Weimaraner dogs disappeared in our area that very same weekend. As for horses, I rode only two between the time I was born and the time I turned 19 years old. The only reason I started going to horse barns at all was to hunt for good-looking girls!

In my entire childhood there were no hamsters, birds, snakes, fish, or insects placed in glass tanks for hours of observation by a curious scientific mind. There was one exception.

In anticipation of the annual July 4th festivities, my mom often cleaned several used glass peanut butter jars with metal screw on lids. Using a nail, we punched small air holes in the lids and added a handful of grass and twigs to the jars. The time before sunset was occupied with playing ball, swimming, or bicycling with our red, white and blue streamers flying in the breeze. The family feasted on the standard picnic fare. In the pause before fresh strawberry shortcake made its entrance, my sister and I would dance around the growing darkness trapping lightening bugs as they lit-up the night with their glowing tails. 'I got one' would be heard repeatedly as we trapped the mystical creatures in the jar. As we stuffed fresh July strawberries and hand whipped cream covered with sugar into our mouths, we marveled at the silent explosions of light coming from the trapped bugs. Even though I never owned a horse, somewhere in my early years, a connection with animals was forged and then lay dormant for more than a decade.

Much like all children, I had dreams. I wanted to become a world-class swimmer, then a SCUBA diver, then an oceanographer, then a construction worker, then a photographer, then a truck driver, then a horseman, and finally a veterinarian. As I look back, I laugh as I imagine a *Divine finger* trying to steer this haphazard, seemingly directionless life onto a specific course.

Along the way, people with good intentions either directly or indirectly got in my way. I heard things like: "Ya gotta be smart to do something like that," "Who do you think you're kidding?" "Nobody in your family has ever done anything like that," and "Don't embarrass your family." Guilt was often heaped and piled with words as well as facial expressions, hand gestures and body actions. The result of that discouragement could have been devastating for my dream but I had, as of yet, no dream to snuff. I was just experiencing life so it rolled-off me like a distant wolf howl for the most part. Sometimes, though, I thought that maybe they were right. Maybe I just wasn't suited for anything. My self-esteem was tiring of playing defense but no plan was showing to improve it.

My friends and family, thankfully, had a different attitude than all the naysayers. They had a more laissez-faire approach to child rearing and I was allowed to aimlessly pursue life as I would an endless buffet table from the time I left home. As I bounced around from one profession to another trying them on for size, excuses were made that could have suppressed my self esteem further, but it didn't. Rather the opposite occurred. I noticed that I was really good at everything I did but I just wasn't clicking with one thing. Nothing held my attention for very long and I didn't feel passionate about the various things I tried.

For example, our football team was undefeated for three years in high school, but I didn't want to play football after that. I dove underwater in Florida caves and Atlantic shipwrecks at night, but I didn't want to do it every day the rest of my life. I could park an 18-wheel, semi-truck on a dime but I had no excitement about mile after mile of highway rolling by. I felt like I had the skills to literally do anything, but I hadn't found the one thing that I really wanted to do.

As I was searching for what would really make me happy, two things happened. First, I became a friend, then husband, to a woman who had absolute faith in me. She opened my eyes to the wide range of possibilities for my future that I hadn't even considered. She propped-up my self-esteem and nurtured it, giving me the confidence to believe in myself as much as she did. For this I am eternally grateful.

The second thing that happened to me was that I became aware of life as a process that always sought to be neutral. Life wasn't *for* me or *against* me. It just existed with no favorites. No invisible force kept me from what I wanted – in fact the only thing in my way was me! From a position of neutral I learned that all things became possible. In other words, any position away from neutral prevents life from unfolding the way it should. Fear and scarcity such as worry and doubt set up roadblocks. Blind ambition or forcing an outcome creates energy that repels things and prevents you from seeing all possibilities. Everything good that has happened in my life came from being neutral and allowing. It also came from very hard work and focus but always came from a neutral state, which allowed all the possibilities and changes in life's direction to occur.

As I think back over the decades of my life, I can pinpoint when my direction changed and good things came to me. Those times were always associated with being happy, being in the moment, and not worrying about "what if."

It is with horses that I came to know what neutral means and how to just exist in happiness. I was about eight years old and my family – mom, dad and sister Judy – had gone to Texas for a week. Dad had a business meeting there and we stayed at a ranch. There I met "Patches" and the love of horses had me for good. At my next birthday party, I unwrapped a stuffed horse and named him "Patches." I slept with him every night until an embarrassingly older age.

I was about 13-years-old when our family again took a trip this time to Seattle, Washington. We stayed near the Mt. Rainer National Park and I rode a horse high-up on the trails. I remember that I did not have fun riding. To me it was boring except for the moment when somebody's saddle slipped and they went rolling off the left side of their horse and almost died sliding down into the ravine. I could just imagine all the straight-faced horses laughing at these foolish humans. Back in the barn however, you couldn't pull me away from the smells and the presence of the horses in the stable. I spent as much time as I could there doing nothing but, well, just being. Next to riding Patches in Texas, I was probably as close to being neutral, in the moment, or just plain happy, as I had ever been. Yet I was a city kid in a horse barn – it didn't make much sense.

Is there a Divine plan that connects everything? I don't know, but I do find it interesting that nearly 50 years later, my favorite horse to work on in my practice is named Rainer and every time I see that horse it reminds me of that happy time near the Mt. Rainer National Park when I was 13.

## HER LOVING ARMS

*My mind spun while I tried to assess the damage to my body. I had just vaccinated the horse and drawn blood for a Coggins test with no problem. When I started to float his teeth the horse objected to the point of requiring sedation. I injected the medication and he settled down nicely. I was just standing there talking to the trainer not really paying attention to the horse as I waited for the sedation to take effect. As I turned back to the horse to insert my float into his mouth, the drugged horse opened his mouth and lunged as hard as he could at me.*

*The large, chestnut gelding's teeth landed hard in the center of my chest and I was thrown against the wall. I quickly peeled back my layers of goose down, chamois shirt and T-shirt and saw the skin of my left breast bruised and torn. My mouth hung open in shock as I stared at the horse and then at the owner whose eyes were wide. The sedated horse just stood there with his head hanging low, asleep and in another world.*

*I gathered myself and left the barn hoping that my day could continue without a trip to the hospital. I pulled into a parking lot to do a quick self-assessment and as I peeled back the clothing, saw purple, red, green and yellow bruising, but the bleeding had stopped. I decided to continue with my day, though very sore.*

*My next stop was a pony boarding barn run by the sweetest little lady named Ruth. Ruth was in her mid-sixties and lived alone on the farm. She had been the person who had started every adult horseman in the area when they were children, now she was teaching their children. Everyone loved Ruth and she loved them and lived for her ponies. Ruth called me the "young, handsome vet" and whenever I arrived on her farm for a visit, her energy was equal to a puppy wagging its tail.*

This day, I pulled into Ruth's barnyard and she met me with worried eyes. She saw something was wrong before I had taken a step. This is how horsemen are. They are connected to everyone and everything around them and can sense when something is wrong.

I quickly told her about the attack trying to brush it aside. Her eyes gazed in worry at my chest and she demanded to see it. Honestly it was a mess, but with a quick glance, then a touch, she took action. Against my protest, she left me in the barn and disappeared inside the tack room. I waited as I heard doors and drawers slam in response to her search. Soon she emerged carrying the items she deemed necessary for my healing. After shedding my shirts, Ruth skillfully started to wrap a horse bandage around my chest incorporating a large ice pack over my wound.

To pass the wrap around me, I automatically lifted my arms into the air like a compliant patient as she stepped close to me. With her body pressed against me, the small woman stretched her loving arms around to pass the wrap from one hand to the other. She lingered, and then I felt the hug.

She finished the job in silence with two more turns around me then taped the ends securely. I suddenly realized that this woman, loved by so many, was very alone.

She smiled and her sense of accomplishment was beaming as she stepped back saying, "That will help you a lot."

*I knew her love had helped me that day and maybe I had helped her a little bit as well.*

*Ruth was a tough angel to all who entered her life including me. I had several calls to her farm over the next year and she always inquired about my chest. The day I heard of her sudden death from an asthma attack I was in shock.*

*Ruth helped so many with their journey into the world of horses and placed her loving arms around so many, including me and I'll never forget her.*

# CHAPTER 1

*— Swing and a Miss —*

# CHAPTER 1

There were many times in my life I had what I'd call a swing and a miss in choosing a profession. Though I considered my time in Ohio to be the beginning of my life with horses, we can't appreciate it unless we go back years earlier to New Hampshire - Hanover to be exact.

The autumn day was crisp and brilliant. My dad, mom, my sister Judy and I had driven in our Ford Country Squire from Chappaqua, New York to visit Dad's alma mater, Dartmouth College. Mom packed a tailgate picnic including fried chicken, corn bread and deviled eggs. We drank fresh apple cider and lusted for the homemade spiced oatmeal raisin cookies we called "oatmeal rocks."

Dad was a 1936 graduate of Dartmouth then continued after graduation to earn his business degree at Dartmouth's Tuck School of Business. He then went on to Harvard to attain his degree in law and became a corporate lawyer for CIT Financial Corporation in New York City.

My grandfather on my father's side also attended Dartmouth and later became an executive at Westinghouse. Somewhere in the 1920's, Westinghouse sent him and his family, including my dad, to live in Japan for three years.

These two immediate ascendants of mine were definitely movers and shakers and, quite frankly, smart. It doesn't end there.

We are blood relatives of William Jewett Tucker who also attended Dartmouth in 1861. He later became a doctor of theology and in 1886 became the minister of a church in Amherst, Massachusetts. Dr. Tucker published an article accommodating Darwin's theory of evolution in his church as well as support of other "radical" views. Because of these views, the congregation charged him and four others with heresy. His case made it to the Massachusetts Supreme Court where he was acquitted of all charges. The mark of this case was later a part of the famous Scopes Monkey Trial.

Later, Dartmouth begged Dr. Tucker to become the President of the college, and in 1893, he accepted the position. Through his efforts, he earned the appellation "founder of the new Dartmouth" from which the college today, and its graduates, are benefactors.

I was in Hanover buying anything dark green with a white "D" on it. I was a natural for Dartmouth and we were attending the football game so I too could learn the spirit of the campus. Few years in my childhood passed without Dartmouth football games and the Dartmouth Choir singing all the college songs, which I memorized and sang constantly. *Oh, Eleazar Wheelock Was A Very Pious Man...,*

*The Hanover Winter Song, The Twilight Song,* and, *Dartmouth Undying.* Decals covered my windows and pennants adorned the walls. I was a natural for this place.

Unfortunately as it turns out, my ancestry, memorabilia and song memorization were not enough for me to get into Dartmouth. They apparently were looking for grades. The rejection letter arrived in the mail and a stunned silence enveloped the house for days. Now what? After that, the other college rejection letters hit our mailbox in rapid fire, as if I was standing in front of a firing squad. The first bullet did not kill me, nor the second. I hung in there helpless to stop the carnage as the last bullet of college rejection ripped into me.

Ninety percent of my high school went on to college and my guidance counselor was going to make sure that all of his students got there. He had been working on me for years, sending me to remedial classes, hoping something said there would spark a flame in me. While I was sure that Dartmouth was where I was going, I really had no desire to go to college other than I was supposed to go. That's what my family did – they went to college. There was no direction in my life but there sure was the pressure of what the rest of the family had achieved academically.

The counselor called me to his office after he had heard of my embarrassing number of college rejections and said he had been working with a college on my behalf. He said that if I were willing to leave before high school graduation they would accept me into a summer experimental program. Because I was looking for rescue at this point, and it was my one and only offer from any college, I accepted. In mid May, I enrolled in Ohio Wesleyan University in Delaware, Ohio. It was two weeks before high school graduation.

My time at Ohio Wesleyan didn't last long. While I loved the computer class and had been working with computers since 1969, I hated being in the computer room until the wee-hours of the morning trying to find the one line of code that made a pointless program work. Of course, I didn't know that Bill Gates was doing the same thing almost at the exact same time somewhere on the other side of the country. The difference was that he loved computer code and was passionate about it. I wasn't.

If my life were a campfire, at this point you would be giving up on me ever catching on fire. Combustible lighter fluid and matches were being thrown on wet wood and wet leaves with no hope of catching a spark. I borrowed a friend's 350cc Honda dirt bike and drove 30 miles outside of town and found a cemetery. Alone I sat asking the spirits around me what I should do. They decided the best thing for me was to lower the temperature to about 35 degrees and have a fun bike ride back to the dorm. With a frozen body, I decided this school wasn't for me. I sat alone trying to warm-up and think warm thoughts. Then I applied to oceanography school in Jensen Beach, Florida.

The Florida Institute Of Technology had just opened up a new school called The School of Marine And Environmental Technology. We called it FIT-SOMET. Because they were new, they accepted anybody and I was just somebody with money to pay for tuition. Now this school was fun. Diving underwater was an integral part of oceanography and I already was a SCUBA diver certified by the YMCA, the first official certification program. I virtually lived underwater during high school. I watched all of Jacque Cousteau's shows and read everything he wrote. I drew pictures of an underwater house I was going to live in one day. Being underwater was a major spark in my life and that is where you could find me on any summer's day I could get away from work.

My life seemed to be nowhere near horses. I was learning oceanography and photography at FIT but I never saw a horse while I was in school there. I hated the class work and still didn't understand why I couldn't do well on tests – even when I knew the material. I was ready for a change after only a short time at the new college, but that change was almost made for me by a seemingly innocuous event unrelated to my education near Christmas in 1972. I almost became a felon.

I owned a 1969 blue Ford Econoline van that could hold plenty of people and therefore had become a "friend" to many. When Christmas break came, about six people asked if they could split the gas and ride north with me. Sweet deal I thought! Before sun-up, we all piled in the van and were in good spirits as we drove north to our homes. Interstate 95 did not exist yet in south Florida so I was heading north on US Route 1 and US Route A1A along the East coast of Florida between Ft Pierce and Melbourne. These were two lane, back roads that transected every small town between Miami and Jacksonville. In the micro town of Grant about an hour north of campus, I got pulled over for speeding in a 35 MPH zone. The police officer checked out the "long hairs" in the van and forced me to drive to a house on a back street of town. It was still dark and I was in no position to argue with the officer. Everyone in the van kept very quiet.

I was instructed to leave the van and follow the officer. My nerves were jumping out of my skin. We entered the house where I was warned to mind my manners. He said, "The judge will see you in a minute. Have a seat." I sat in the living room of this house on high alert. I'd seen this in a movie once and I didn't like the ending. My upbringing kicked in as the judge entered the living room in his bathrobe and sat at his desk. The words out of my mouth were limited to "yes sir," "no sir," and "I'm sorry," along with a final "Thank you sir" as I shelled out $35 cash and he wrote something in his big ledger. There were no computers or even a recording of my license. Just a warning not to speed in his town ever again or I would be in bigger trouble.

I crept up the coast and dropped the first batch of friends off in Washington, DC and made it to New York without further incident.

On the trip back to Florida I picked up everyone at their homes. Two of my so-called "friends" were really happy. They retold the story of the near bust we had experienced and thanked me for being so cool.

"Why?" I asked.

They laughed and said, "We didn't want to tell you and we're glad you didn't know, but we had a suitcase full of drugs, man! That's why!"

I started to rethink my life with these "friends" right then and severed my ties quickly. It became the start of me never really trusting people.

Aside from this close call of becoming a felon, there were some good things that came from this school. For instance, my love of photography really began here.

I had never been officially instructed in photography until I had been required to take photography courses as part of the oceanography curriculum at FIT-SOMET. My dad had taught me about photography when I was 12. I can still hear him say today, "The larger the number, the smaller the hole," as he taught me how the f-stop aperture of the camera worked. I had joined the eighth grade photography club in 1967 where I developed my first roll of black and white film. I learned at a young age about the mystical process of turning light into a paper memory. Dad and mom bought me my first real camera while I was in Florida. It was a Nikkormat film camera, which wasn't the top shelf but was better than 90 percent of the other cameras out there. I went everywhere with that camera and still have some of the photos I took back then. I think my parents were hoping they were getting some smoldering embers from my campfire and they were fanning them in hopes of erupting flames. All I knew was that I was very happy taking photographs.

I also learned at FIT-SOMET advanced diving techniques including deep diving (150 feet), night diving, salvage diving, and cave diving in northern Florida. "Awesome" and "beyond belief" were descriptions of my diving experiences. Hovering above a sunken ship in the black of night in the Atlantic Gulf Stream off of Palm Beach, not knowing if sharks were close at hand hiding in the dark was thrilling. Hovering in crystal clear water in the Devil's Eye cave in Ginnie Springs with no light other than our lamps 90 feet below the ground with only one way out is still indescribable. These lessons in self confidence and self esteem were absorbed, filling me with all the necessary gumption to make this work and it almost felt like I was getting somewhere - that is until marine microbiology.

Suddenly I was again lost in the classroom. It wasn't due to lack of effort, but it was those pesky little exams. One day I was taking an important exam in marine biology that had really big words made up of smaller words that alone I could remember, but in combination proved too much for my word mating skills. They all looked the same to me. I looked at the paper and wrote simply, "Out to lunch" for each question and handed it in.

I felt defeated. My roller coaster had been high the weekend before as I dove in the ocean and photographed everything in sight.

Now, as the professor called out the grades to the class, his deep voice cleared, then said, "And finally, the lowest grade of the exam belongs to the student who wrote out to lunch for his answers."

I packed my things and loaded them into my van. I said good-bye to all the friends I had made there and then wrote a brief note to my mom and dad. It said, "I'm leaving Florida. I'll let you know where I am when I get there." I sealed the envelope, stamped it, and slid it in the outgoing slot in the local post office. I got in my van and headed north to Ohio, the only place where I still had friends but was far enough away from my family in New York to give me some peace. I was embarrassing my family and myself. I felt alone in the world.

I pulled into Ohio where I had lived less than a year earlier and quickly learned that many people thought I had died. Someone who looked like me with the same first (spelled Jeff) and last name had drowned canoeing so when they saw me walking down the street, many screamed or became overwrought. A friend said he had seen a ghost of me once, drenched in water, walking down Main Street. It was fascinating to see and I was touched that people who had known me for only a year had thought enough of me to mourn -- or hallucinate!

I quickly learned that being broke is not fun. Other than being with a few friends, I wasn't sure I belonged in this town, and was down to my last few dollars. I had sent a note to my parents that if my son had sent to me, I would have hunted him down and kicked his butt. They weren't going to send me any money. I needed a job.

An opening was available at the paint manufacturing plant outside of Delaware, Ohio where I was now living. It was Friday and I went to their employment office. I was clean and wearing my good clothes when I entered the office. My attitude was positive. The man showed me around and said if I wanted the job I could start by driving the loader that would fill the railroad cars. The tires were 10 feet tall and a little intimidating.

I loved driving anything, as my childhood sand box filled with graders, loaders and dump trucks could attest so I said, "Sure thing," and I was hired.

He said, "Report here on Monday, 8 am sharp."

That weekend I celebrated and got my funds down to maybe $10. I was on time Monday and reported for work. The foreman said, "You never was hired, long hair. Get going now and don't come back."

I was numb and drove my van around for a while. Then, as if someone else was steering the van, I drove up a long driveway into a large Saddlebred horse farm. I walked up to the person in charge and asked for a job. I was desperate.

"You ever work with horses before?" he asked.

"No," I replied, "but I'm good with my hands and I like to work."

He said, "Wait here and let me get the boss lady."

After a while, a well-dressed woman entered the room followed by her Afghan dog. She and her dog had a unique bond and they even looked similar. I immediately did not like her or her dog, but that wouldn't be important. I was getting a job as a farm grounds keeper and would not be with the horses. At that point, I didn't care because I needed the money.

I was teamed up with the old man in charge of the grounds but I wasn't sure if he liked me or not. I was another pair of hands that he needed for spring cleaning. He had me only doing the things he really did not want to do.

I remembered from my short stint in a horse barn at the age of 13 that good looking girls usually hung around barns and with the security of a steady job and the assurance my parents were not coming to get me and kick my butt, I started to go looking for some female friendship. A special note needs to be said again about my non-interfering parents. They never judged me but loved me where I was and for that I am eternally grateful.

A tall, lean brunette with green eyes and a brilliant smile caught my attention in the barn. Her name was Candy and she was working hard with a wound up Saddlebred as I screwed up my courage to start talking with her. In no time at all I was in love, but she was only interested in a friendship. Candy kept me on a very long leash, but I thought, "Hey, at least I'm on a girl's leash!" I'm so dumb sometimes.

Candy invited me into the barn for lunch and I would stay to watch her put a tail set on a horse. This is unique to the Saddlebred breed and is required for showing them in competition. I started to spend time with Candy in the barn as well as driving together to and from work. She was living with another man but I was falling deeper in love. I still remember her smile but of course I had no chance with her beyond friendship. My introduction to horses in Ohio lasted only a short time but it was pivotal in setting into motion what still inspires me today.

It would take two defining moments before my true passion for a lifetime with horses would really gel. The first was a Johnny Carson show and the second was witnessing a bizarre medical treatment of a horse.

Many people remember watching The Johnny Carson Show back in the 1970's. It was really worth staying up past 10 pm to watch. I loved the variety of guests, especially when he had one with wild animals. The guest would be chatting away while the animal just did what animals do – which was often something unexpected and unpredictable such as slither across Johnny Carson's desk and onto his lap. Johnny's reaction would have me laughing so hard I cried!

This particular night's show was in the spring of 1973 and the famous singer, Dean Martin, was the guest. He sang a song then sat down with a drink in his hand and, obviously a little tipsy, tried to hold a conversation with the host. I was going to turn the show off because it was boring but I became frozen on the couch with Johnny's next guest.

"Our next guest," Johnny announced, "takes photographs of people's halos. It's called Kirlian photography." Please welcome..." Out came a man in a suit who sat between Johnny and Dean, two wealthy and iconic men. He was a nobody really, but he soon became the single most important man in my life.

"Mr. Martin, would you mind if I place your hand in this light proof bag?" Dean, a little tipsy, said, "Sure thing. Are you going steal my ring while it's in there?"

The man said with a serious tone, "No, Mr. Martin. I'm going to pass 10,000 volts through your hand which will cause your auras to glow and will be recorded on the photographic film in the bag."

Johnny, as well as everyone else, was bent over laughing with tears flowing from our eyes as Dean desperately looked around and started to get up to leave. He was pulled back down into the chair where he took another long drink of the amber fluid in his glass. Sweat started to form on his brow as he said, "Te, te, ten THOUSAND volts?"

The man, waiting for a break in the laughter, reminded everyone that volts don't kill, amps do, and what he was using wouldn't hurt anyone.

In an act to assure Dean, the guest performed the process on himself. The Polaroid film developed instantly and he revealed his finger auras. He then did Dean's auras. "We often see a broken ring aura with alcoholics," the man stated as he peeled the paper off of the film. Sure enough, there were broken rings.

Everyone was laughing but I completely tuned out all noise and thought, "Wow! Energy off the finger tips!"

The next day at the barn near lunchtime, I went to find Candy. While I waited, I visited a large, chestnut gelding who was afraid of everything. Eyes bugged and nostrils flared, the big horse stayed in the back of the stall snorting at me, the stranger. His neck went vertical and his head tilted slightly sideways, his bulging, right eyeball staring deeply into my face reading every nuance of every expression I made. The chains that Saddlebreds wear around their artificially raised hoofs made ominous noise as he pranced in place, almost like a rattlesnake warning me to stay far away. Since I'd just realized we all give off energy, I wondered if this horse could sense that. Horses are notorious for being able to sense fear in those around them. I wondered if this horse could also sense calm. I stood in the stall doorway and focused on relaxing completely. I released a long breath out of my nostrils and slowly lifted my right hand palm down. I focused on emitting calm energy off of my fingertips toward this horse.

To my shock and amazement, the horse dropped his head, slowly exhaled in response, and then advanced toward me gently touching his nose to my fingers. I was thrilled and overwhelmed. I had made my first real connection with a horse and I was hooked. This incident plays in mind almost every day as I encounter new horses and it had a huge bearing on my eventual decision to become a veterinarian.

The second life-changing event occurred one day when I was outside raking leaves on the farm. The quiet morning was split with an explosion. I froze for a moment and then started to rake again. "Ka-Boom!" again but this time I vectored the sound to determine that it was coming from the indoor arena. With the third explosion, I abandoned my station and went to the arena to investigate.

I entered the front of the building that led into the observation area. Sitting there was the trainer and assistant trainer. In the ring alone was a wide-eyed, vertically necked blood bay horse walking freely about the ring. I asked simply, "What's going on?"

The trainer said, "This mare has colic."

I asked, "What's that?"

He looked at me finally recognizing that I was the outdoor guy that didn't know anything about horses other than the cute girls that worked with them. He informed me that colic is an upset stomach in the horse. "When they get it," he said with a slight arrogance in his tone, "they like to roll to ease the pain. Unfortunately when rolling, they sometimes twist their intestines into a knot and if that happens they die. To prevent the horse from rolling, we throw ash cans, cherry bombs, and M-80's to scare them into running."

He had quite an arsenal of explosives in his bag. He looked at the horse and saw she was pawing the ground. This was something a horse with a bellyache would do just before getting down to roll. The trainer withdrew a round, red cherry bomb with a long green stem and lit the fuse with his lighter. Arching the sparkling colic treatment into the air toward the horse, his aim and timing was perfect. Just before hitting the ground and about 10 feet from the horse, it exploded. The sound inside the arena was so much louder than what I had heard outside with thundering echoes bouncing off the walls and ceiling. The horse leapt into the air and ran with all her might. Eyes almost popping out of her head and nostrils flared, with each full stride of her long hind legs, a short staccato eruption of gas escaped her anus. "That'll fix her guts!" the trainer said with some laughter of contempt.

Something unexplainable rose in me. My guts and my conscious screamed that what I was seeing was wrong. I felt that horse's fear and pain, but there was nothing I could do to ease it. I quickly turned and left the building. I went to find Candy but she said that she was leaving for Massachusetts the next day and would stay in touch. This crushed my dream of being with her and I soon found myself heartsick and just plain sick with what was later determined to be a bad case of mononucleosis. It was time for me to go. I had $24 dollars cash and a full tank of gas as I left Ohio and returned to New York. I crawled into my childhood bed at my parents home and fell asleep for three days.

When I finally woke up I realized that I was going to remain with horses somehow, someway. I knew in the deepest part of myself that they would be my passion and my life. I had finally found my purpose and direction.

## PUT HER DOWN DOC. SHE'S AS GOOD AS DEAD.

*The dark winter's evening sky had enveloped the land and my regular day was done. My bones were warming and my stomach was filled with great food. This evening would be perfect if I had no emergencies and I could snuggle into my warm bed piled high with a feather comforter. My long day wasn't over as the answering service called about a colic 45 minutes away.*

*Risking this being interpreted wrong, I have to say that I enjoyed working on colics. For me it was an easy diagnostic exercise with concise parameters that could be interpreted accurately. My goal was to determine if the horse had a medical colic or a surgical colic and I had developed a reputation at Cornell's emergency clinic of being not only accurate, but because I sent them in early, about 90 percent returned home after surgery – an excellent outcome.*

*I drove through the evening with confidence in my abilities to quickly assess this horse's situation and return home with another successful outcome. Helping my confidence was the trainer who* had called me. He was a professional with experience and I knew he was calling me about a serious colic. He knew the difference between a minor issue and something serious and would never have called me if it were other than serious.

I pulled up in front of the long, pole barn with a roof higher than in most. I gathered my equipment and briskly walked in the cold, January air through the dimly lit barn. The trainer stood in front of the open door and without looking up at me said, "Put her down Doc. She's as good as dead."

I quickly looked in and saw a familiar picture of a blanketed horse lying down in the middle of the concave floor. She was covered in a thin layer of bedding shavings collected in the material of the blanket and hair of her mane from rolling about in agony. Her eyes were glazed and distant and the nostrils flared. The odor of sweat mixed with the smells of urine, manure, and old shavings penetrated my senses and added dramatically to the scene before me.

"I've tried everything short of beating her to get her up," the trainer said. "It's no good."

I knew this trainer would have tried every way he knew to get the horse to stand. If she wouldn't there was really nothing that could be done other than relive her misery. I started back toward the truck to get my euthanasia solution but almost like you see in a cartoon, I felt an angel on my shoulder speaking clearly in my ear. "Wait! You went to Cornell. What did they teach you there? They taught you to do a full exam. Go back and do a full exam!"

I turned on my heel and went back to the horse that was now moaning. I bent down with my stethoscope and listened to the heart. The rate was only slightly elevated. I could hear a moderate amount of gurgling in the abdomen and my training started to tell me that this wasn't a serious colic. "What was it?" I asked myself silently. My mind was evaluating the situation as I decided I absolutely had to get this horse up to examine the other side.

To get her up, I first needed to get her blanket off but it was twisted tightly about her body. I unbuckled everything but the last thigh strap was very tight. I struggled to release the tension and after successfully releasing it, laid the blanket to the side and gently tapped her back with my toe.

The mare sprung to her feet, did a full body shake, and walked over to her hay and started to eat. The trainer and I both stood with mouths dropped open in disbelief as we alternated our gaze from her to each other and back to her. I was the first to laugh out loud as we both realized that this very sensitive National Show Horse thought she was dying from a thigh strap that was too tight and pinching her leg. Talk about a Drama Queen!!

The trainer involuntarily made himself small with bent knees as he quickly walked out of the barn in complete embarrassment. I turned to my shoulder and thanked my angel.

# CHAPTER 2

## —*I Need Work*—

# CHAPTER 2

June in New York had always been the best time in my life. The cold, wet rains of spring were replaced with what we in the Tucker family called "top down weather." Dad would drive his family for "sunset drives" in the Metropolitan, a very small, yellow and white, car with a black canvas convertible roof, that we called "The Putt-Putt." Mom would occupy the copilot's seat, wearing a babushka that flapped stiffly in the breeze. Judy and I would stuff ourselves in the back seat where the square foot area was the size of a shoebox. We never knew if a trip would cause fighting matches between us or we would laugh uncontrollably. We would often stop at Carvel for a soft serve ice cream cone – it was a wonderful time.

June also marked the end of school as everyone broke from the rigors of learning to a life of fun in the sun. During the later years of high school, I worked either as a golf caddy or on the town crew cleaning storm drains and operating a jackhammer. These jobs had early quitting times and there was still plenty of time to go to the beach or SCUBA dive. I had enough money and life was good.

This year, however, was a different June. I was no longer in school. This was not the start of summer vacation. Rather, it was the start of my life as a man and a horseman. I needed to find a place to work and live. The rose-colored glasses I always wore in June were set aside as I squinted against the afternoon sun.

I had left Ohio two weeks before and was feeling better about my life having a clear direction now. I left my parent's house late in the morning and drove to an area where I knew there would be horse farms, but I had no plan. I was scared but I always had a bed and a meal with dad and mom.

I drove to Mt. Kisco and then out to the hills of Bedford. It was close to afternoon feeding time at a Thoroughbred breeding and training farm off of West Patent Road when I pulled into the long barn driveway. It was the first farm I looked at for work.

The long white barn with green roof and trim was symmetrical. A back-to-back feed room and a tack room followed five, back-to-back stalls for a total of 10 stalls and 2 rooms. These made up one half of the barn. After a break through the middle of the barn, there were another six, back-to-back stalls. The total of 22, 12x12 foot, stalls were encircled with a rideable shed row and everything was contained within the barn walls. This was the training barn where the young horses were saddled within the stall, mounted, then ridden out into the shed row and trained.

Behind the barn was a half-mile training track to gallop and condition the horses. Between the barn and track was a circular pen made of chain link fence. Within this pen horses were lounged, or if they had an injury, were turned out for fresh air but had limited space to ensure they would not re-injure themselves.

Earlier that day, the pen had another use. An employee high on drugs had taken a horse into the pen and started to beat it. Walt, the trainer, caught him and fired him on the spot. When I drove up, Walt and the owner, Mrs. Trotter, were standing by the pen discussing how to handle the duties being one man short. As I approached, their looks of concern turned from their matter of being short-handed to me. I introduced myself and said that I was looking for work.

Walt was a former jockey and exercise rider. His short stature had weathered hands that were constantly bringing cigarettes to his ever-trembling lips. When he talked, his words would be mumbles. His body lurched sideways as he walked. He was a strange man with physical injuries only he and his wife knew about, but he knew horses - Thoroughbred horses specifically - better than he knew anything else.

Mrs. Trotter was a dominating and imposing woman. Hips that moved with authority supported her towering six-foot stature. Her facial expressions could be kind with understanding eyes and a melting smile, then in a blink of an eye, would turn into a sharp tongued lashing of a person's soul cutting to the depths of her opponent until she emerged the victor. Her thick glasses frequently traversed down her nose, exaggerating the size of her eyes, to quickly being clutched in one hand and shook at the person she was talking to emphasizing her point. Her agitated state could always be determined by the degree she fiddled with her ever-present glasses. She was as strong an ally as one could have, but also a woman who would say without hesitation what was on her mind.

Mrs. Trotter of course took command of my impromptu shed row interview. Walt took a step backward.

"Have you any experience with horses?" she asked.

I lied; "I know how to put a tail set on," remembering watching Candy do the same. That, at a Thoroughbred breeding and training farm, was useless as I later discovered. Her question though had another purpose. She was digging to see if I had character that was better than the last drug head that had just beaten one of her prize horses. I told her I was from Chappaqua and my dad was a New York City lawyer hoping she would realize I was from a good, hardworking and honest family.

I was hired on the spot, to start the next day. I was earning $80 a week, working five-and-one-half days a week. The job also came with my own two-bed, one bath apartment. Walt didn't say anything, but I was overjoyed!

Bill, the farm manager met me at 7 am on my first day at Trotter Farm. Bill is a little hard to describe but eccentric probably suits him well. His mind was always somewhere but not always with the person he was talking to at the time. His eyes twinkled and his lean body moved with little grace, jerking with hesitation as his thoughts took him one way, then another. In mid-sentence sometimes he would end his conversation with you and suddenly just turn and leave. Bill drove a 20-year-old Willis Jeep pocked marked with rust, and he often ground the gears that sounded like fingernails on a chalkboard to almost everyone on the farm.

Bill had a tendency to answer questions rather cryptically, which was sometimes a challenge for me. "Can the horses be turned out tonight?" I would ask.

His answer simply would be, "The Yankees are playing tonight."

Many a time an answer like that would stop me dead in my tracks as he walked out of sight without another word. I'm sure he never thought twice about it, but sometimes having to guess what the heck he was thinking would keep me up at night!

For the first time, I really felt like I was doing what I was supposed to in life. I had a job – and not just any job – but one where I spent all my time around horses and learned more with every new day.

Bill led the way. "You'll be working here at the training barn," he said. "Chris and Robert will make sure you know what to do here. I'll be back at ten or so to show you your apartment."

We walked inside and found Chris, a redheaded woman who looked like she was all business and acted like she was the boss. I saw through her tough skin right away into her kind heart. She was my introduction to a type of female that I describe as a "barn girl," my highest form of compliment to a woman. A rough exterior with hardened hands but a warm heart and a willingness to work well beyond the limits of a normal person. Chris was always riding horses or cleaning tack. She often pitched-in to clean stalls if there was nothing else to do. She never complained and took one-quarter tab of Bute, a potent horse painkiller, for menstrual cramps or cracked ribs, and kept smiling.

Robert was a black man who had been with Mrs. Trotter for a very long time. He lived with his wife and two sons, Sam and Mike, on the farm. He was a workhorse and could effortlessly manipulate a pitchfork full of manure like a gambler could flip cards and he loved to laugh. He knew his job, and his worth, and was understandably a little miffed that an educated white boy was in his barn.

As if he were saying, "Here, educated, upper class white boy, let's see if you know how to use a pitch fork," he showed me the tools and pointed me in the direction of my first stall.

I am fully aware that all animals, including humans, look the same with the skin removed, but this was 1973 and only a decade after race riots in America. I soon realized the difference between whites and blacks was deeper than skin color and there were many layers of prejudices and incorrect assumptions to get through that flowed both ways. I discovered prejudice was all in our minds and I soon went to work on creating a good relationship between Robert and myself. Why? Because we can learn and grow from everyone we meet and at this point, Robert knew a lot more than me about working with horses and I was humbled by that.

In a short time, Robert and I became friends enough for him to invite me over for Sunday dinners where I tasted collard greens for the first and last time. He loved to barbeque and I enjoyed the time I spent with his family. I became friends with his sons, Sam and Mike, as we played softball with other farm kids in a paddock where cow flops served as the bases.

The next two years became the best two years of my life up to that point. I became addicted to work, mowing pastures on my day-off just because I enjoyed being outdoors with nature and horses. I would rise at three in the morning and walk one-and-a-half miles to arrive at work by four. Chores were done about 10 am, and I was off until 2 pm, when afternoon chores started and then finished by four in the afternoon. Often I would stay during the midday break and repair fence or clean the hayloft. I never thought about what

I was paid versus what work I performed. I never thought about vacation. I was always on-time for work and I can't remember taking a sick day. That is the difference between doing something for a paycheck and doing something you love – it never feels like work!

The physical size of Trotter Farm was larger than I thought that first day and it took several months before I understood the lay of the land. There were two divisions: Mrs. Trotter's farms and Mr. Trotter's farms. I worked for Mrs. Trotter who had the training barn, the pony barn, Newell's barn, the old folks home and the "other" barn. Mr. Trotter had his barn where the stallions stood and the horses in training at Belmont Race Track.

There were about 100 horses total on the farm and that number ballooned to 300 with visiting brood mares during peak breeding season. On average, over the years, seven stallions stood with five Thoroughbred stallions at Mr. Trotter's barn and two at the pony barn including a world champion pony stallion. Breeding and foaling season was over when I arrived in June that first year and the farm was full of nursing foals.

My job in the beginning was simple: I cleaned the 11 stalls on the west side of the training barn stripping out all manure and urine using a metal, 5-tined pitchfork and rake. I then added lime to the urine soaked clay floors and shook apart wheat straw using the fork until the stall was covered in a bright, yellow fluff. Then I added three flakes of hay, cleaned and filled the water buckets, raked the dirt shed row, and swept clean the wood planks laid between the dirt shed row and the stalls.

In the summer, the horses stayed in the stalls during the heat of the day and were turned-out overnight when it was cooler. In the morning, Robert and I would muck the stalls into the shed row. He was on one side of the barn and I was on the other and we paced ourselves, but he was always faster. The mares with foals trashed the bedding and soaked everything with a lung scorching ammonia urine smell each day. Every mound of manure and wet spot was heaped into a pile just outside the door, then the exposed clay dirt floor was raked clean and a layer of hydrated lime was spread over the remaining urine to absorb the odor. Over time this layer became crusted and the pitchfork tines would stab and catch the thick, cardboard crust. It would peel back into a thin two square foot piece weighing 20 pounds or more. I would vainly attempt to balance it on the end of the pitchfork as I lifted the one piece trophy, carefully rotated on my heels, then lifted higher to place it on top of the 5-foot high pile of straw and manure outside the door. It was these small games I played that helped me through the morning. It was boring and hard work especially during inclement weather, yet I was learning very small lessons that proved essential to my growth as a veterinarian.

The next part of morning chores involved the starting of the ancient red Dodge, medium duty truck with dump body attached to its frame. With a door that barely closed and windows streaked with barn dirt, cracked mirrors, hard un-powered steering, and an engine that somehow turned over every time there was enough energy left in the battery, I carefully backed into the opened door at the end of the shed row. This truck often went to the service garage for repair.

One day after the vet came to the farm and performed a castration, I took the discarded testicles and placed them into a bag. I drove the truck downtown and directly into the service bay. The Rhodesian Ridgeback dog performed guard duty and was always covered with patches of grease from lying in the junk piles. He eyed me carefully as I exited the cab and looked in the office for George, the owner of the shop.

George was somewhere between ornery and just plain mean where I was concerned. He obviously saw me as a nobody from the farm, which I was at this stage of my career. On this day, George looked up from his desk, identified me, and gruffly said, "What now?"

I calmed myself and then said, "The truck's got no balls! You need to find out what's wrong and get its power back."

I turned and left him with his quizzical look transforming into one of frustration as I walked back to get my things. I removed the testicles, looked to make sure the dog was chained up, then threw them under the truck and left. My trick didn't help the truck any, but obviously liking the joke, George became a little friendlier to me after that.

After backing the truck up the shed row of the training barn, I would tumble out of the cab and walk back to the manure piled outside the first two stalls. Then fork load by fork load, I would pitch the manure into the truck. Sometimes when horses were left in due to bad weather, and the loads were twice the normal size, Robert and I would double-team and together lift larger than normal, urine soaked piles into the truck. Using a time-tested strategy of pile placement within the dump bed, we could get an amazing amount of waste in a load. To really fill it, I would leap onto the tailgate and climb on top of the pile, brace my hands against the ceiling rafters, and perform a stylish "poop shoveler's dance." This packed the load even further allowing us to add more before declaring the load full. Robert's dance always had more soul than mine and shoes didn't last long on this job. Though we never fell off or broke our legs, there were times when we almost did. OSHA (Occupational Safety and Health Administration) did not exist and if it had, we probably would not have complied with any safety regulations in order to get the job done as quickly and efficiently as possible.

The truck had farm tags that allowed us to travel anywhere in town on farm business without insurance or inspection, hence little was spent on maintenance. On a daily basis we slowly drove the truck out the long drive and traveled one-quarter mile down the road and turned into a dirt path that led to the manure pile that was out of sight from the road. Turning in the small wooded area and avoiding trees, stumps, and wet sink holes; we backed into position and lifted the dump body high to watch the load of manure slide out the back.

Sometimes a well-packed load would catch and not slide off. To correct this, I would get out of the truck and with a pitchfork, pull-off half the load by hand. This difficult task was always made worse by either a downpour or a 20-degree blizzard, which seemed to happen with some regularity.

With the load off, I popped the clutch and tore out of the manure pit. As the dump body gently lowered itself, the truck would hit every dip or rock violently swaying the truck sideways effectively throwing off any remaining bits of hay and straw. Then, as fast as the truck would allow me, I would drive it hard back to the barn, shifting the gears without the clutch, and repeat the process one or two more times that morning. The last load was always mentally easier than the first.

While I was at the dump, Robert would rake up the shed row, leaving a beautiful herringbone pattern in the dirt. Water buckets were then cleaned and filled. When all was done, we went to get the horses from the paddocks. This was the part of the day I really loved. While I did not know it then, I attribute this time of learning and observing the horse as the greatest part of my veterinary education.

Chris, Robert, and I would walk about 100 yards up a hill to catch the mares and foals. There were ten pairs and sorting them became an art form. Realizing who went first and how to avoid being kicked was essential to continuing work without injury. Bringing a mare and foal out through the gate, without letting the rest of the fly fearing, hungry, feral mares out to run freely about the farm, taught me that calmness and leadership was essential. I was new to it but with Chris and Robert's help, while not always successful, I did okay – and I learned quickly. The horsemanship skills I use today in my veterinary practice can trace their roots to these beginnings where I was not only challenged with hundreds of different horses, but I was blessed with great teachers who cared that I got it right.

Now it may not seem like much, but 100 yards is a long way to lead a horse. In the relatively short amount of time spent turning out or bringing in horses from the far field, I began to form the horsemanship skills necessary to follow a lifetime of work with them. Today's vets magically go through high school, college and then vet school. There is talk of shortening this path as veterinarians are becoming glorified technicians. Whenever "old timers" get together to discuss horses and veterinary care, the subject of how veterinarians today are not horsemen always comes up. If it was up to me, I would require all candidates for vet school to leave the academic world and spend two years cleaning stalls and walking horses 100 yards every day. It is this practical hands-on experience of being with and observing horses that gives you a larger understanding of their problems and essential care. It taught me valuable lessons I still use today.

One lesson I learned was just observing the movement of the horse and how much it can tell you about their health. I clearly remember watching the hind legs of the horses ahead of me as their hocks rotated outward with each step. Later, in vet school, I would remember this as it helped me to understand that the hock is as much a rotational joint as it is an opening and closing joint. It became essential to my understanding of hock disease such as bone spavin. Two years of almost daily walking and watching twenty-two horses, with or without foals, up and down a hill, became an integral part of my understanding of leg movement, balance, symmetry and pathology. Within a short time, I could pick out a subtle asymmetry of the very early stages of a lame horse at a walk.

I was always told from my first day at Trotter Farm to turn the horse around and have it face you before turning it loose either into a field or back into its' stall. This was (and is) the proper way to do things to avoid the horse kicking you as it goes by.

I was also taught that when leading two horses together, take each lead rope and pass them through one hand so that the one end of one rope exits from your hand in one direction and the end of the other rope exits out in the other direction. This way if the two horses decide to take off on you, all you need to do is squeeze the ropes together with either your one hand or with both hands. The horses will then only be pulling against themselves and not dismembering your hands and arms.

Leadership among horses is learned and encouraged. With foals, the first mistake people make is to allow the foal to follow the mare without a lead. What this teaches the foal is to be a follower. In addition, he is not taught that mutual respect is necessary in a human world. Horses are herd animals and allowing nature to take its course, most become followers with only a few leaders. These following foals can become dangerous as well as unproductive in their lives.

To avoid this, we always haltered our foals and lead them in front of the mare. By simply doing this we developed young horses that respected us and became more cooperative when being taught more advanced lessons such as accepting a saddle.

My first two years at Trotter Farm were formative in more ways than I can consciously realize.

# A SAD DAY ON THE NEW FARM

*The young family had just bought their farm in the spring a month ago. 5 acres of woods surrounded by more forest. The house was brand new and moving boxes still littered their driveway and garage.*

*I drove up the drive forking to the right onto a dirt path leading around the house. I saw their two horses standing in a clearing in the woods. The couple and their daughter came out of the back door to great me.*

*"Thanks for coming out Doc," the woman said as she led the way to the paddock. "Our sorrel gelding has stopped eating and is acting depressed."*

*She was right. He didn't look like he had colic but stood quietly with his head lowered below his top line looking at the ground. He wasn't relaxed nor was he fretting and he showed no interest in food. Depressed seemed to be the best description. She slipped the halter and lead on him as I looked around at the surroundings.*

*The trees were mostly deciduous: maple, cherry, and oak. A few pine trees scattered themselves about. One electrified wire* made up the fence and it was strung through the woods claiming about an acre. Tree stumps remained from the clearing process and limbs and branches were placed into several tall piles. The trunks were cut and stacked for winter firewood. There was no grass or any evidence of hay nor was there a barn or even a run in shed.

I asked, "Tell me about this pasture," as I started my exam of the horse.

"We just moved in a few weeks ago," the man said proudly. "The first thing we did was string a wire through the woods to make a place to turn out the horses. Plenty of shade and storm protection."

I moved my stethoscope around the abdomen, lungs, and heart. Nothing including the temperature was abnormal. My mind started to struggle with what could be causing this horse to be so off with no clear physical signs. The man continued to describe the making of the paddock.

"We let the horses settle in and last weekend I started to cut the trees down to make a clearing," proudly showing his efficient thinking. "We plan to pull the stumps and then plant some grass seed."

He had moved his family into a new house, his primary goal, and had proceeded to make the wife and daughter happy by moving the horses soon thereafter even though he really had no good area prepared for them.

I lifted the upper lip of the horse and blinked at the surprise I found. The normally pink mucous membranes were muddy brown. My heart sank as I started to prepare my approach in telling them that not only was the horse going to die, but also it was their fault. The resulting effect on the family would last a long time and like every vet, I dreaded being the one delivering the news.

"Your horse's kidneys are failing," I started. "They are being plugged with debris much like a kitchen strainer gets clogged and the water can't pass through." There was silence.

"What can you do?" they asked. At this time, a vet at Cornell who I knew had just published the toxic effects of red maple leaves. There was no known treatment and I told them this.

"Red maple leaves? What do you mean?" they asked. I continued to explain that when fresh, green maple leaves start to die after a branch is removed from a tree (as in a storm causing a branch to fall or after being cut down), the wilted leaf becomes toxic to the horse. It causes the red blood cells to burst. Their contents clog the kidneys, which leads to acute renal failure. The muddy brown gums are the telltale sign and the rapid damage causes the horse to die quickly.

The father understood. By cutting the trees down and keeping the branches in the paddock, he had killed this horse. Making it worse was substituting the tree leaves for forage in the effort to save money in giving hay.

*The sad day ended for me with euthanizing the horse followed by a long drive home. I never saw that family again and I suppose they sold the other horse, which had not been affected yet, ending their short life with horses.*

# CHAPTER 3

## — *Death Comes Swiftly* —

# CHAPTER 3

Anyone starting a career in anything knows the first year or two consists of a steep learning curve and working with horses is certainly no different. Lessons are learned by observing other people doing things and following what they do. As you have probably already learned about me, I do nothing easily. Rather than learn from mistakes of others, I often learn from my own and sometimes those lessons were life threatening.

In 1973, we always had a halter and lead rope on to do everything with a horse. We also always wore a helmet when riding. We always played by the rules and with little exception, had no injuries. Those in charge, who knew so much about horses, also knew that while they are beautiful creatures, they could also be very, very dangerous. When you think about it, a horse weighs 5 to 10 times more than a human. You wouldn't let me run into you full-speed as it would definitely cause some injury! Now imagine one of these horses running into you. Odds are you wouldn't live through it.

Horse owners, trainers and vets often work around horse's legs and frequently run the risk of getting kicked. To understand the danger, think about me swinging a baseball bat at your head with all my strength – scary isn't it? A horse's leg is much heavier and more muscular than a bat and can swing at the same speed, fracturing bones, causing organ rupture, internal bleeding and death. I have known people who have succumbed to all of these.

There are rules that are important to abide by, to lower this risk, so you can work around horses everyday without fearing for your life and I learned many of these early on. However, today's horse owners break these rules constantly and are injured and killed daily and I understand how it can happen. In my first year alone, I almost became a statistic three times – it's a wonder I survived at all, even though I'd been taught better. I never said I was smart.

It's easy to look back at times you did something and barely cheated death. Invariably you come away humbled and feeling very stupid – after all, you knew better, right? Has it ever happen to you? Well, it happened to me!

Sassabe Star was a pregnant, chestnut mare living in the first stall beyond the break of the barn. She had little affection for humans, as her life had become a baby factory. Most people who are what I call "city folk" fail to understand that all animals have memories, opinions and feelings. They aren't just objects. They have personalities and emotions and that will catch-up with you if you aren't careful. Another thing city folks don't realize is that animals, bigger and stronger than a human, can kill you without blinking an eye. It is easy to understand the danger of Grizzly bears and sharks, but not a sweet and affectionate horse. They would never intend harm, right? Wrong! This was the day that I realized that I, too, was a city folk.

She was my sixth stall of the morning and the barn was quiet. As anyone who works with horses constantly will agree, you can never let your guard down, but we all do. The horse that will kill you is probably your own – or one you work with every day. This is because even though we know to constantly be aware, we get complacent, bored or just lazy and we forget. We forget that a horse is the size and weight of a small automobile and can mow you down in an instant. We forget those four legs we see and work around every day, can crush your skull.

I was in her stall cleaning it and I broke the rules – and it wasn't just one rule I broke, it was three, specifically: no halter and lead rope; the horse between me and the exit; trusting a horse I was familiar with. I was complacent and not connected with the horse. Add a touch of irrational fear in the horse and the disaster was ready to unfold. Horses frequently get 'spooked' and panic. It could be from a loud noise outside, a small bird fluttering through the barn, or it could be something they totally imagine! Either way, they panic and are gripped with irrational fear and you never know when it might happen.

I was in the diagonally opposite corner of the stall to the gate and was digging out some manure in the corner. I had closed the gate so I could go to that corner without the horse running out. I was not listening to, nor paying attention to, the feral brood mare and she decided to communicate her displeasure with me.

Dust and straw arose as she started to scramble. I wheeled myself around and placed my back into the corner of the stall. The mare had her head in the far corner by the stall door and her long back with enlarged abdomen was sunk lower than normal toward the ground and her hind end was facing me. I watched as if the whole scene was in slow motion. Her hips lowered some more and the muscles of her hindquarters tightened. Her hocks and stifles were flexed and her weight now shifted to the front limbs as she rose slightly onto the tips of her hind hooves. The first kick was imminent.

I was frozen in place. My mind went blank as I searched for options. The stall walls were smooth and 10-feet tall. I could leap up grabbing the top edge and swing my body up over into the next stall. I doubted my athleticism and worried what the surprised horse in the next stall would do. I quickly ruled out escape over the wall. What was left then?

I had heard that time can slow when you are about to die. The purpose of this I learned that morning when I decided to do something I would have normally thought impossible with the amount of time left before the hind hooves punctured my body. It was something leaders do when faced with impossible odds. I cleared my mind and became calm.

I had also heard that your life would flash before your eyes before you die. I can tell you that this is true as well. Within one second of real time, I had replayed everything significant that had happened in my life in sharp detail. I have not heard why this happens, but I can assume that everything in life has a purpose. I believe that if you have lived a good life, the remembrance can give you inspiration to take action so you can continue your life rather than paralyze yourself with fear and inaction. If however your life has been bad, then you will not take action and you will allow events to unfold that will kill you.

I decided that I had more to live for, but if I was going to die, I was not going down without a fight. I firmly grasped my pitchfork, forced a loud, harsh toned, growling scream as if I was an angry bear attacking, and swung the wooden fork handle across her buttocks. The mare instantly swung her head to the right and did a quick two-step to avoid the wrath of this crazed human. I saw an opening to her left and in one giant step lurched towards the stall door past her still cocked haunches and bounded onto the dirt floor falling face first to the ground. The mare sank into the back corner of the stall as I gasped for breath and felt my heart pound through my chest. Our eyes met and we both knew the outcome was a surprise to us both.

Though I'd barely escaped with my life, I learned two very important lessons that day. The first was that I was not scared of horses. The second was that I was committed to giving my life to them. Fear can keep you from being effective when dealing with animals large enough to kill you. You have to come to terms with this fear and get past it. I also learned to never let my guard down and constantly stay connected especially around horses I know well as they can, and will, kill you.

My two years at Trotter Farm was my testing ground and my future plan to be with horses seemed to be unfolding flawlessly. I had learned so much about them and had developed a solid work ethic as well. Physically I was in great shape, looking lean and well muscled as I had unloaded trucks and wagons of hay and straw, unloaded railroad boxcars of oats, and ate little, living the bachelor life.

With my focus on horses, I was not spending too much time underwater now and my SCUBA equipment stayed stored at my parent's house and was eventually sold. Occasionally I would go out on their boat but being underwater had been replaced with the peace of watching horses graze in a field. However, another passion started to compete with horses and that was photography.

I set up my bathroom as a darkroom. I covered the windows in light blocking aluminum foil and I created lightproof seals for the door. I thought photography could become my higher income profession and I wanted to give it a try, even though horses had my heart.

I applied to Brooks Institute of Photography in Santa Barbara, California and was placed on their waiting list for acceptance almost a year later. Again, it looked as though schools were just a business looking for money and they really did not care if I was academically acceptable. I had dinner with my parents and broke the news to them. I laid out their financial commitments and sat back proudly with my thoroughness.

My poor parents, once again. Their point of view was simple. While not being negative and fully understanding that I needed a higher paying skill, they reflected on my track record and drew me into their compassionate conclusion. "Okay," they said. "This is the last time we will pay for your education. If you quit, you're on your own."

I should have guessed that was coming and they were absolutely correct in their assessment. My parents had seen nothing but my happiness during the time at Trotter Farm, but they knew it was a dead-end street with no advancement potential. They believed in me and knew I was better than a manure shoveler. My past failures academically and socially still haunted me. There was nothing to run from, yet I strongly felt the need to run away. Why not California? It appeared risk free. Maybe, I thought, distance would ensure my success.

In May 1975, I packed my 1974 Dodge van for a month long journey out west. I built into the back of the van a bed that could fold up on the side. I also made a set of music speakers with woofers and tweeters and a crossover network that stood about three-feet tall and weighed 30 pounds each. I secured a Coleman icebox and stove into practical positions and filled in spaces with boxes of things such as clothes and food. My bright yellow, "Canary Cottage," as my grandfather called it, was ready for the drive across America.

Six-months earlier I had found a German Shepherd mix at the Millwood, NY SPCA. He was given a clean bill of health in the free vet's exam that came with the adoption that day and I decided to call him E-Z. A short 24-hours later I returned to the same vet with my new friend now with projectile diarrhea. I was angry that he was so sick after receiving an exam recently. Even though the vet did nothing egregious, I was left with a feeling that I had been dismissed because E-Z was just a pound-dog and I was not wealthy. Nobody likes to be treated this way and it became another lesson I would never forget in how to deal with animal owners with respect and dignity.

I took E-Z home and cared for him as if I would die if he did. I know he sensed my love and even though he had been given-up by someone as a puppy, and he had no reason to trust another human, he seemed to forgive me and my species, rested himself in my arms, and as we slept together that night, began the healing process that cured his diarrhea and bonded us for life. E-Z followed me everywhere on the farm but his greatest love was to plop himself into the passenger seat of my van and either look out the window while I drove or sleep in the sun. It was before sunrise when E-Z and I headed for my tightly packed van on our way to a new adventure in California. I drove the van out of the pony barn driveway and away from my first home and away from my parents. E-Z went to sleep in the seat.

Pru, a friend of mine in New York, had given me two books before my westward trip. The first was *Travels With Charlie* by John Steinbeck. The story was about one man's travel across the country with his dog Charlie and the adventures they had. The second was a journal of blank pages where I could write my thoughts.

My first two weeks were boring. I made several stops on my way to the Mississippi River where I said hello to different people, but every stop seemed disappointing. Maybe I was looking for a friend who would say, "Geoff, this looks like fun! Can I join you?" It didn't happen. Slowly I realized I had no friends, at least no one who was looking to do something different in their lives.

E-Z was a great friend but was not a great conversationalist. Once I reached California, my first order of business was to find a place to stay. I was not looking to rent in town so I traveled the areas where there were horse farms. I entered an area called Hope Ranch, which was a community of exclusive homes, many with horse farms. I found a beautiful place overlooking the Pacific Ocean and drove in.

Just like I had done two years before, I had no plan but I had an expectation of a positive result. Was I scared? Yes, but I also knew what I wanted. I found a farm and a girl named Cathy who stabled her horse Timberlein there. She lived in one half of a duplex in return for taking care of the horses for the owner. I told her I was looking for a place to live in return for working on the farm and somehow, by the end of the day, I was moving into the other half of the duplex.

Cathy was beautiful and I was falling in love immediately. Having plenty of experience in the stupid department, I tried not to show it and kept my thoughts to myself. It was easy because Cathy showed no interest in me other than being friends.

The farm was beautiful too. It was created and built by the architect owner who lived there with his wife and gorgeous daughter. The house was a beautiful California style and looked nothing like what I was used to on the East coast. The views of the ocean, with the Catalina Islands in the distance, were spectacular. The house sat on top of a cliff. Paddocks and an outdoor arena lay between it and the six-stall barn, the duplex, and another guesthouse that was empty. I soon came to the conclusion that everything and everyone in California was beautiful. It was without exception.

My classes in photography started at 8:00 am sharp. I soon was becoming proficient in the dark room where there were at least 20 stations. I bought a 4x5 inch view camera and tripod. This type of camera was used one hundred years ago and I'm sure you have seen them in old movies. The photographer, with his head under a light proof cloth, would tell everyone to hold still, and then an explosion of light would ignite the material on the flash pan and a puff of smoke would envelop the area. While our flashes were now electronic, the principles of tilting the lens and the film plane to compensate for distortion were the same. Each shot was meticulously planned. Lighting was metered and the picture content was framed. One shot was taken, then the film removed from the camera and replaced with another piece of film measuring 4 x 5 inches and another shot was set up. It was a very long process.

We also studied studio lighting, the positioning of models, chemistry and legal matters involving the capturing of people's images used for commercial purposes. There were tons of great stuff to learn, but I quickly became uninterested. Again the horses and I would find each other.

Cathy's dad was a high-ranking polo player in Santa Barbara and I soon was visiting the polo fields in Carpinteria about 30 minutes southeast of Hope Ranch. Cathy and I attended the games and I would start to pitch-in cleaning tack, cleaning stalls and rolling the countless leg and tail wraps after they were washed. I learned the ins and outs of polo and soon found myself grooming for the games. I was even allowed to wrap their tails before the game knowing that if I did a poor job and it fell off, I would owe a case of beer to someone. I offered to exercise the polo ponies in the morning because the players couldn't consistently do this during the week. They readily agreed.

This is a good point to say that I had never really ridden a horse before. Starting Monday, I was going to exercise 15 to 18 horses by riding one horse and ponying two others along side. If this sounds simple to you, realize that not all of these polo ponies were calm trail horses. They were just the opposite with high temperaments and minds of their own, on what they were, or were not, going to do. So it took me much longer than it might have an experienced rider to get everyone exercised.

I woke-up in the very early hours of the morning and in the dark found Oaxaca, a horse that I fed and cared for on the property in exchange for a color television for my apartment. Once he was fed, I then drove 30 minutes to the polo field and again, in the dark, tacked up one horse, gathered two others, and headed to the dirt oval track. I would do a turn at the walk, then trot, then gallop enough to make them breathe a little hard. I would return to the stables, untack, brush-off all evidence of tack from the hair coats, and repeat the process until the five or six sets were back in their stalls eating their morning feed. While this doesn't really sound like much to a horse person, you need to realize that I did this all before my 8 am classes. I loved it and was obsessed about being with horses.

The Santa Ynez Valley is on the other side of the mountains from Santa Barbara. Getting to it requires a drive through a pass that, when on the other side, takes your breath away. The yellow and pale green rolling hills are dotted with large bushy trees that appear to float over the ground. Many horse farms are located here, and on occasion, Cathy and I would travel there to witness a hunt where horses would chase the scent of a fox. One of the obstacles the horses would be required to jump was a chicken coop filled with live chickens. That one was fun to watch and photograph, as the potential for disaster was ever present.

I loved Santa Barbara. The easygoing way Californians lived was a sharp contrast to the high-energy of New Yorkers. The weather was always perfect. There were miles of beaches.

The land was beautiful and there were plenty of horses. I was not homesick and there was absolutely nothing I could think of that would make me want to go back East.

One day, a family moved into the empty guest house and it was apparent the man was an equine veterinarian. His name was Dr. Munson and he was starting his practice in the area. How perfect was this I thought? Here is someone who could really teach me something about caring for these beautiful animals. I soon made room on my plate to include any time I could with this man. My first steps toward becoming a veterinarian were the encouraging words by him and other veterinarians as they answered my questions.

The first equine veterinarian to encourage me was Dr. Wilson at Trotter Farm back in New York. He was retired then and came to the farm to do the herd health and the newborn exams. With his experience and seniority, he taught me to not take life seriously and to joke a lot. Dr. Simpson became Dr. Wilson's replacement on the farm and while he also had energy and a great work ethic, his influence on me wasn't appreciated until much later.

It was therefore Dr. Munson who truly became my first mentor in equine veterinary practice. Today most practitioners have help in the truck, but back then Dr. Munson worked alone. His wife kept the books and did the office duties as my wife did years later when I started my practice. Any chance I could get to ride on calls with him

I took, but I didn't have the passion for veterinary medicine yet. My agenda was just to learn more about horses at this point, not to become a veterinarian. The idea of me ever going back to a real college was off my radar screen.

One day, I found Dr. Munson in the wash stall of the barn with a horse in the crossties. The horse was very sleepy looking and the crossties were fighting to maintain their integrity as they equally held the weight of the heavily sedated horse. The vet was a very quiet man and methodically moved with deliberate measure. I asked what he was doing and it took a moment before he responded, "I'm castrating this horse." He didn't say no when I asked if I could watch, so I kept my distance while he worked. In little time the job was completed and I thanked him and left.

I had seen castrations before and they were usually done in a dark and dirty stall with one man holding the horse with a lead rope and a twitch twisted tightly on his nose. The horse was sedated but not enough for cutting off his testicles so the twitch was necessary to keep him still. Nonetheless, the colt would usually try to take a few sideswipes with his hind hoof at the vet. Here though, Dr. Munson worked in a clean and well-lit environment and he worked alone. Also unique was his use of a human leg crutch placed under the horse's chin to support the head while the operation was performed. It looked clever to me as this one-man show did what other vets needed two or three people to do.

On another day, I was hanging out with Dr. Munson as he stocked his truck. His wife came out to tell him there was a colic case that needed his attention. I was about to ask where his stock of firecrackers was but I decided not to ask. I just got into his truck and rode along. I had only been with horses for a few years but I had seen several colics. All had been medical and were treated with all sorts of concoctions including just walking it off. Today, as we pulled into the small farm located behind the house, he muttered, "Oh no. This doesn't look good."

This horse was very uncomfortable. Dr. Munson took out his stethoscope and performed his exam. He passed a stomach tube, administered medications, and talked with the owners. What impressed me, and has stayed with me, was how he treated these people. He was straightforward and polite but also compassionate. He took his time explaining to the owners what was going on. At this point I didn't understand exactly what was wrong, but I knew this was a colic that concerned him. I have modeled my approach to clients in my own practice based on this one event.

We climbed back into his pick-up and as we were just rolling out of the driveway, Dr. Munson turned directly to me and soberly remarked, "That horse isn't going to make it."

We drove home and I don't know what we talked about. All I knew was it was the first horse I knew that was soon going to be dead and there was nothing that could be done about it. Numbness entered my mind. I didn't realize it then, but it was my first experience of self-preservation. My mind takes bad experiences with horses and dumps that memory by the time I reach the end of the barn driveway. In my years as a veterinarian, I quickly realized that if I internalized the pain and suffering horses went through, I would be committed to a psychiatric facility in short order. Looking back I clearly see this day with Dr. Munson as my first detachment of the outcome because to do otherwise, would have turned me into an ineffective veterinarian.

Dr. Munson went on to develop a large and successful equine practice and then became a professor at a prominent Veterinary College. I have seen him at a few meetings where he lectures on very practical things. I have twice thanked him for his mentorship but I don't think he really remembers me. The short time I had with him helped form me, and my style of veterinary care, though at the time, I didn't realize it.

My stay in California was soon drawing to an end. With all that I loved about it, I needed to leave. Photography was fun but was quickly becoming a chore. "Working" as a photographer did not inspire me and was certainly not something I was passionate about. I spent every free moment from three in the morning until I went to bed with horses. I had bought the book *Lameness in Horses* by O. R. Adams. This was the bible every vet used to learn detection and causes, as well as treatment for horse lameness. I couldn't pronounce most of the words, but still I would fall asleep reading it. I memorized the drawings and pictures.

I was becoming exhausted as I worried about what my parents would say when I told them I was quitting college yet again. I couldn't help but feel like a big failure and my self-esteem was tanking. Three strikes at an education and God only knows how many strikes with girls that went nowhere. I needed some alone time so I walked from the farm to the empty lot next door, and sat down on a stump in the woods.

My mind drifted and I allowed it to. Often clarity comes from letting go. E-Z ran away from me and down the path that led to the clothing optional beach below. He was a regular and I had plenty of time for him to make the rounds and greet whoever was there.

I never fell asleep but I have no recollection of anything between the time E-Z left and his triumphant return. His tongue hung out as far out as possible, dripping gooey saliva over my lap as he nudged me back into reality. Panting heavily, his clear brown eyes penetrated mine as if to say, "Hey, I'm back. Are you all right? Wanna throw that stick for me?"

In my hand was a long thin stick. It was not the type I would select to throw for a dog and I really don't remember getting this stick. I looked around wondering why I had it.

When I looked down I saw a patch of sand at my feet and a drawing of a horse's head I had made with the stick. I have no recollection of doing it, but apparently my subconscious knew more about what I wanted than my conscious mind did at that point. I smiled from ear to ear. I shouted, "Come on E-Z. We're going back to New York!"

## IF YOU DON'T PULL OUT MY HEIFER CALF ALIVE, I'M GONNA KILL YOU!

*It was a warm summer's day and the grass and trees were green. There was little humidity and the temperature hung in the upper 70's with a light breeze.*

*I was on my rounds of the farms my boss had set on the list. Hen scratch on a torn piece of yellow lined paper with his faint words echoing directions in my head "Go into town, go left on The Mariposa Road then right on The Grist Mill Lane and so forth. He always added the word "The" in front of the name of the road.*

*I was about an hour late getting to this farm where a cow had been having difficulty delivering her calf.*

*I was fresh out of vet school and looked forward to my life with horses. But until I was earning enough to pay the bills in my own practice, I had joined a nearby general country practice. We treated cows, dogs, and cats as well as pigs, sheep, goats, rabbits, and yes, a horse or two. I would work all day then drive 44 miles home and change into clothes void of the barn smells. I then went off on my own horse calls until late at night.*

*It was on this brilliant summer day in upstate New York where I learned about confidence. I had tied the tail back, cleaned up the cow's perineum, and with my arm lubricated, I entered her birth canal. My hand and arm gently twisted and my fingertips ended against a wall of twisted uterine tissue.*

*I pulled out and stood up and faced the cow's owner. He was a no nonsense scruffy looking professional herdsman. He showed contempt as he starred at this new, wet-behind-the-ears, veterinary graduate. "What about her?" he said with point blank expectation.*

*I was excited because I knew exactly what the problem was and how to deal with it, though it was my first. "Your cow has a uterine torsion," I exclaimed with pride.*

*His face screwed up as he shot "What? Say it in English!"*

*"The calf has twisted the uterus along the birth canal. The opening is closed and there's no way the calf can get out," I flatly explained.*

*"All right, what can you do for her?" he said quickly getting to the meat of the situation.*

*"Oh, it's simple. We'll do a Plank In The Flank." My confidence was based on the very clear discussion of this approach*

*I had recently learned in my lectures at Cornell. Though I had never done one, it made sense to me. My professor though never told me what would come next.*

*"Your gonna do WHAT? What the Heck! Where's your boss? Plank In The Flank? Who's ever come up with that?"*

*His rants would have gone on but I felt more confidence welling up in my gut. I told his assistants, who had been watching silently nearby, to find a 16 foot long 2 by 6 inch wood plank and take it along with the cow up to the grandmother's house where there was a large grass lawn. Apparently my barking of specific orders instilled some confidence, at least in the help.*

*We assembled ourselves on the flat grass-operating field. I placed my rope around the cow's neck and passed the end through the metal quick release loop on its end. Positioning the loop where the withers would be on a horse, I took the rope rearward along the cow's backbone just a few inches, then turned the rope at right angles away from me and down along the cow's right side. Recovering the end of the rope underneath the cow, I brought the end up her left side and slid it underneath the rope at her backbone effectively forming a loop of rope around her at the girth area.*

*I repeated this forming of a loop around the cow's body just in front of her hipbones. The remaining rope I proceeded to extend rearwards about 3 feet behind her. With someone standing in front of her and holding her by the halter, I proceeded to pull my end of the rope behind her as hard as I could. My pulling caused the two loops of rope around her body to compress her sides. This cow, like dozens of others before her, just dropped without objection to the ground and then fell to her side.*

*It wasn't just any side but the correct side because I had guided her. This part had been important because my next step was to place the end of the 16-foot board on top of her abdomen just in front of her hips. I would stand on the end of this board that was resting on her abdomen. My weight would apply downward pressure trapping the calf in the uterus. The 2 men would then roll the cow over to her other side while I kept the calf inside the uterus in place effectively untwisting the uterus. However, if she was placed on the wrong side then all we would do is twist everything tighter.*

*I conducted all to their positions while I mounted the board. Another thing my professor had forgotten to tell us was how hard it was to balance on top of this mass. Beach Boys songs about surfing leapt into my mind. While I struggled to balance, I ordered the men to "Roll the cow!"*

*Slowly the process commenced. I danced and regained my balance. The cow groaned but did not struggle. Completed, I jumped off my perch and positioned myself behind the lying cow.*

*As I inserted my hand, the owner came up behind me and calmly but clearly said, "If you don't pull out my heifer calf alive, I'm gonna kill you!"*

*My fingers at this point touched the calf's nose through a now opened birth canal and the calf very much alive bumped me back. I turned my head and looked at him and said with a cocky attitude, "What if I pull out a live bull calf?"*

*Without a blink of an eye he said, "Then I'll just maim you."*

*By now I had my hands around the calf's legs and was pulling out the bundle of life. I had no worries about him maiming me, and my cockiness got the better of me. So I said, "What do I get when I pull out a live heifer?"*

*He paused, than said, "I'll buy you a case of beer."*

*I made my last effort to pull the large heifer out and she breathed her first breath. "Make it two cases!" I said.*

*I never got a drop of beer from this farmer that summer afternoon. I gained from him though an understanding of human behavior and a feeling that I had chosen the right profession.*

# CHAPTER 4

## — *Kentucky Bound* —

# CHAPTER 4

I traveled north along the California Coast. I need to admit one thing about that part of the country. It is absolutely beautiful, but I come from the East Coast where windows never shook. Earth tremors were common in California and to this day I use it as the reason I left. After all, there were plenty of horses in California and the land and girls were beautiful. I really had no reason to uproot again but my inner voice and the Divine Plan had me driving East, back towards New York.

Before I had left Trotter Farm, I had become friends with Steve and Betsy who were co-workers there. They had moved to Paris, Kentucky and were the managers of a large Thoroughbred farm. I had plans to stay with them and their son Jeremy for a week and look for work there. I was not ready to fully return to New York and face my parents.

Thoroughbred farms in Lexington are nothing short of stunning. Steeped in tradition, their long black fences partitioning fields of lush green grass dotted with mares and foals give the timeless appearance of royalty in the equine world. I wanted to be a part of this. All I had to do, I thought, was drive onto the farm, present myself, and I would have a job. It had always worked in the past so why not here?

Apparently there were many people like me looking for work and I was rejected repeatedly. So, I changed my approach and aimed higher, looking at the best farms in Kentucky. It worked at Spendthrift Farm, the largest Thoroughbred farm in Lexington. They were not really looking for help, but I had a letter of recommendation from Mrs. Trotter and apparently the manager of Spendthrift knew and respected her. He decided to talk with me and then drove me around the farm.

The man asked me what I was looking for as he drove the miles of roads between the barns. Out of thin air, I said, "I'm looking for a job with upward mobility."

The guy nearly drove off the lane when he heard that. "Upward mobility!" he repeated with his bushy eyebrows lifting up to touch his hair line. He thought, then he said, "Because Mrs. Trotter thinks so much of you, I'll give you a chance to prove yourself." He showed me the house trailer next to the training track where I was going to live then took me to the brood mare barn where I was going to work.

Butterflies churned inside my stomach as I quickly became aware that I had my foot in the door of the greatest Thoroughbred farm in the mecca of Thoroughbred farms.

I returned to Steve and Betsy's and we celebrated. Then I made a quick trip home to New York to visit my parents and get my belongings in order.

Two days later I was with my parents having dinner. As always, they were gracious and supportive of me though, as I look back, they had to be hoping against hope that I would stop roaming the country like a nomad and settle on something, anything. It was suggested that I go visit Mrs. Trotter and thank her for her letter. The next morning I drove to Trotter Farm and found her. Upon learning of my leaving photography school and my new employment in Kentucky, Mrs. Trotter turned on her irresistible charm. She paced authoritatively around her palatial, Victorian room leading with her hips, eyeglasses jiggling in her hand as she pointed them at me while emphasizing her words. Eyebrows scrunched downwards momentarily, then her face would brighten as she bombarded me with compliments, softening her prey before she attacked with her plan.

Mrs. Trotter always got what she wanted and she wanted me to work for her. She drove me to the new house I would be moving into. She created a new position she called the 'assistant farm manager' and even pulled Bill over to the side of the road and, with me in the car, proclaimed to him that I was going to be his new right arm. Bill looked surprised as if he knew his days were being numbered. He finally grinned, popped the clutch lurching the creaking Jeep forward and disappeared. Mrs. Trotter though, had done the same and was moving fast in the other direction back to her house. I told her I needed time to make a quick trip to Kentucky.

Her final words were, "Good. Then I'll see you Wednesday."

I had left all my belongings with Steve and Betsy in Kentucky. I quickly said my thanks to them and headed over to Spendthrift. I apologized and explained and they were gracious. The whole trip had me back in New York in three days. I was at Bill's house at 7 am Wednesday morning and I was very ready to start.

My outlook was bright as I was part of management now. No longer did I need to muck stalls for a paycheck. I never felt more powerful than the workers, but I did feel more responsibility, and that feeling was new for me. It was a feeling that, over the years, I struggled with because I have always believed that all people are created equally and given the same opportunity. However, when given a position of authority where responsibility meant making decisions, I soon realized that I was now looked at as someone better than my workers. This is stuff that countless movies have been made of where the laborer is raised-up to management and the friendships are strained and people's heads explode from the pressure between friends and responsibilities. Ugh, I was uncomfortable.

Overcoming this dichotomy was a necessary transition for me. I had to learn to balance management with my principle of wanting everyone to like me. I created a new style of leadership that as it turns out, has worked somewhat well for me. It is based on being firm but fair. While to this day I am usually too soft in making decisions about other people, I have made more friends than enemies. Most remarkable is that this was the start of my true horsemanship skills, though I didn't know it at the time.

This time of my life is filled with stories of my growth as a man and the discoveries of life. If I were a house, I had built my foundation up to this point. Anything built on top of it would be solidly supported going forward and it was my time to create my masterpiece. All that was missing was talent in hammering the nails and laying sheetrock, as well as an eye for color, decorating, and landscaping. This would change dramatically during the next 12 months.

The learning came fast. I would never be as knowledgeable as Walt but he, as well as Bill, became my willing teachers of things that became a part of my future. The lessons learned can be placed into two categories. The first was horsemanship where I learned to not only handle mares brought in for foaling and breeding, but also to saddle Thoroughbred yearlings for the first time. We called it "breaking the yearlings" before the word "breaking" became offensive to so many. Almost 35 years later, I saw a professional (and famous) "natural horseman" "break" a horse using the same methods we used back then.

The second category was veterinary medicine, including preventive medicine, sick horses, lameness, breeding and foaling. In the 12 months I remained at Trotter Farm, I learned more about caring for horses than I ever learned in veterinary school.

One of the most important jobs of the trainer is to detect the onset of an injury before it actually becomes an injury. One of the best warnings a horse can give is to have heat build up in the leg. Heat is a sign of trouble and removal of heat is the priority in prevention or treatment of the lameness. With so many horses in training, it became my job to learn how to detect heat and I was terrible at it.

Walt, with a cigarette dangling from his lips, would stare at the ground and squat next to the horse. His hand would run along the lower part of the front leg. No man would look more serious than Walt as he did this. He would suddenly stand erect and grab the smoking habit from his lips and mumble to me, "Tell me what you feel."

Being considerably taller than the former jockey, I would bend down with more effort as low as I could and place my hand on the limb right where I thought, if there was going to be heat, it would be. My hope was to find any thermal irregularities instantly and proclaim my prowess as a bona fide horse trainer. I stood up and said, "I can't feel any heat."

Walt was always kind with me but his respect for the horse always trumped cordiality. "Are your hands numb?" he asked incredulously. He placed his hand in mine, removed it, and then placed a cup of hot coffee in it. "Can you tell the difference between my hand and the cup?" he asked looking me square in the eyes.

My confidence wavering, I said, "Yes."

Walt always had a habit at this point of changing his face into a van Gogh work of disbelief. His eyes would flutter under raised eyebrows, his lower lip would dash in and out of the space between his teeth, and then he would suck in a lung full of air, and slowly let it out through his nose, as his lips pursed together and his head shook side to side. He would then gently say, "Try again, but this time start with your hand above the knee where its' cold. As you move down, feel the change in temperature and feel the hot spot."

Midway down the back of the cannon bone I felt an imperceptible rise in skin temperature. I did it again to be sure. I turned to Walt and pointed to a one-inch area on the back of the tendons and said, "There."

Walt smiled then said, "Let me show you how to apply mud."

I grabbed the sack made of several layers of brown paper and filled with fine, brown-red powder. This was Bowie

Mud and it comes from Bowie, Maryland. It had ingredients found in no other mud in the world. When mixed with water and applied to warm areas of the horse's leg, it drew out the heat. The horse world is filled with remedies for lower limb inflammation but I have seen few ever compare to Bowie Mud.

Walt showed me how to mix the correct proportions of mud and water and then apply the mud in an upward direction against the lay of the hair to help it stick to the leg. With wet hands, he would smooth the outside while saying, "If you put on too little it will dry out too quickly. If you put on too much, it will fall off."

We always had brown paper lying around the barn because some feed came in bags made of it. Walt tore off a length of paper with the width being equal to the length of mud on the leg. He wrapped one layer of brown paper around the mud poultice. This prevented the straw bedding from sticking into the wet mud and pulling it off. He then cleaned his hands and I put the horse away.

We had another horse to poultice and he let me try. While it wasn't as pretty or done as fast as Walt's, it got the job done. I went to bed that night feeling a desire to learn more. For the first time I was enjoying school.

I had regular duties including creating and maintaining the preventive medicine schedules. It was easier than it is today because there were fewer preventive procedures. Deworming medications were limited to only two classes of chemicals and they came in packets of powder we would shake over the top of the grain. Many horses wouldn't eat it. Understanding the parasite life cycles was knowledge limited to parasitologists in the universities. The idea of medicating for something we couldn't even see seemed like an exercise in spending money with little results. The only reason we fell for the idea was the excitement of our vet, Dr. Simpson, and our belief in him as an honest authority in caring for our horses.

Dr. Simpson was a young, energetic man with a broad forehead and curly brown hair. He was a full, half-foot shorter than me, but his presence always commanded the attention of those around him. With quick eyes, his intelligence would jump from his thoughts into the words he spoke. He was always moving but would stop, turn and look into my eyes every time I had a question. Time would stop as he effortlessly answered. His patience and willingness to help someone like me, someone not nearly as smart or as educated, became a trait I admired. He will never know how much he shaped me into becoming a vet who would love to teach.

When Dr. Simpson marched into the barn one morning holding a box of small, foil-wrapped powders and announced, "We now have a medication to fight worms in horses!" There was no argument from us. The battle of the invisible enemy was upon us. It was clear leadership and an art form that took me years to master.

Walt at Trotter Farm took injections of medicine very seriously. No other personnel were allowed to stick a needle into a horse. With me now in charge of the farms' preventive medicine, Walt allowed me to give intramuscular shots but this was a rare event. Only when a vet prescribed a medication, and Walt wasn't available, was I allowed to administer the drug through a needle placed deep in the muscle of the neck. Intravenous shots were never allowed. Walt placed a fear of giving injections in my mind that haunted me and prevented my efficiency until well into vet school. While he allowed me to learn many things, this was one he had a deep fear for and now his fear was mine.

You have to remember that vets only administered injections back then. The idea that disease could be spread through a used needle was just becoming popular thanks to devastating outbreaks of Equine Infectious Anemia, the disease that the Coggins test would later be developed to detect. But in 1975, the only way we knew to stop the spread of that disease was to become sterile between horses. Individual, use once and destroy, needles and syringes were replacing the small glass jar filled with alcohol and permanent needles attached to glass and metal syringes. Our farm received the best and most modern care from veterinarians who were on the forefront of veterinary medicine. While Dr. Simpson was our regular vet for almost everything on the farm, Dr. Wilson was the expert vet who would attend all foalings, and was always the final word on matters.

Dr. Wilson was an older gentleman, tall and distinguished, well dressed with a sporting tweed cap and a thin mustache. He carried everything he needed in a classic small, black leather grip, the kind you see in older movies of doctors. He was a past president of the American Association of Equine Practitioners, the largest organization of equine veterinarians in the world. He was fully aware of modern techniques, yet during this year of my learning, I saw him use both the old method of syringe use, as well as the modern disposable needle.

Dr. Wilson was kind to me but never took me in as the inquisitive person looking for help. He rather kept me at a distance, assuming that there was no hope of me becoming what he was. While I'm sure he was a good vet, he seemed stuck in the past and believed himself to be above most people. The difference between him and Dr. Simpson was very evident and solidified my determination to become a teacher. It was from this start that I became a student of personalities and I added the good characteristics and actions of other vets I was around to my own, which made me who I am. The lesson from this is simple. There is something to learn from everybody we meet. Conversely, we teach everyone we meet.

I was still the go-to-guy at Trotter Farm for driving the horse van. I was proficient at it and I enjoyed it. I am a visual guy and being on the road gives me a never-ending source of different pictures. The dangers and excitement of being away from home have been reduced to nothing, compared to the era of the stagecoach. Still, there were challenges.

One night going north on Interstate-95 I stopped to pay the toll at the Delaware Memorial Bridge. The truck was a standard transmission. Using a clutch, I would shift through the five gears and split each gear between low and high ranges. At a stop, the clutch would be depressed to the floor, the engine would idle, and I would find the lowest gear needed to smoothly start the truck again from a stand still.

As I pressed the clutch in and passed the money to the toll keeper, the engine abruptly stopped. I attempted several times to start the engine but all it would do is crank without catching. Nearly midnight, I could see the headlights starting to stack up behind me. The toll keeper reached for his phone and called the service truck to push me out of the toll station and over to the side of the interstate, away from traffic and underneath a large, bright light.

Sunny was one of the barn girls from the farm and was with me in the front. We were on the way home from Southern Pines, North Carolina after dropping off horses there for training so there were no horses in the van. "What happened?" Sunny asked. I started my diagnostics. I have always played-around with engines and had been a rookie auto mechanic in my youth. I had rebuilt my dad's starter motor in his Mercury Marquis without any idea of what was inside it. We were both surprised when the motor worked and he was please it hadn't cost him a dime. Then there was the time I brilliantly grounded the negative end of jumper cables on the air filter post of the carburetor. When I attached the cable, the spark set the gas in the carburetor on fire. This started a mess under the hood of the car, which was parked inside the garage that was attached to my parent's house. Disaster was avoided only because the laundry washing machine was next to the garage bay where I was working. I grabbed a towel from the cleaned clothes stack and snuffed out the flames. I figured a ruined towel was better than a burned-down house.

My seat of the pants mechanical abilities have served me well before the engineers complicated things under the hood. The GMC truck I was driving for the farm was built in 1963 and its engineering was primitive. I decided that warm, summer night to figure out what was wrong, and fix it myself.

For the next hour I used the tools from my toolbox and took the carburetor off the engine. Then piece-by-piece, on the ground and under the tall street lamplight, I disassembled the complex mechanical device that mixes the gas with air and feeds it into the pistons for combustion. In the faint light I saw and then felt the minuscule grain of dirt that had clogged the float valve in the gas reservoir that flooded the engine and made it inoperable. I reassembled the device and mounted it back on the engine. I asked Sunny to start the truck as I watched under the hood for anything unusual. With only a short crank time, the engine erupted into life and purred smoothly as I gathered my remaining tools and closed the hood. Sunny beamed as she moved over to let me in behind the wheel.

I was very proud of my ability to work under stress and to diagnose. What I did not realize at the time was the training I was going through to become a vet. Diagnosing and then treating when situations and conditions were not the best should be a part of every veterinary school curriculum.

## AN AFTERNOON FOALING

*Spring was glorious in upstate New York on this particular Saturday as I made my rounds from farm to farm. I was so excited to be a veterinarian doing what I thought I was put on this earth to do. Asked if things could get any better than this, my answer would be an astounding, "No way!"*

*I had an easy day finishing my last call by noon. I headed home to be with my wife Kathy and my 8-year-old son Matt for lunch. Kathy had some afternoon plans and I was responsible for parental duties. A caveat always prevailed in a veterinarian's life. I was a parent but only if my pager did not announce an emergency.*

*When Matt was young enough to be carried on my back in a papoose, I would go on calls with him exploring an injured eye or listening to colic sounds from the intestines. His head would snap from overlooking one shoulder to the other shoulder forcing my body off balance numerous times. His interest appeared intense and my mind started to think of the new practice name: "Tucker & Tucker."*

*When my pager announced a Saturday afternoon emergency, I reluctantly retrieved the message and called the client. What luck! A mare usually delivers her foal in the early hours of the morning but today was a rare afternoon delivery. Of all things a veterinarian gets to do, delivering foals is absolutely my favorite. With my son being able to attend, maybe, just maybe, it would be the spark that would set him on a course of becoming a veterinarian.*

*When I arrived I quickly determined that the foal's front legs were folded back and it would be stuck without intervention by me. I quickly prepared the mare and my equipment as Matt stayed where I told him and watched intently. We were in a converted dairy barn. Removing the pipe stanchions where the cows would usually stand had created an area about 10 feet square. Boards on three sides were used to contain the mare in the open area. There was fresh bedding where the mare, laying on her side, was trying to push out the baby. Her hindquarters faced the cement aisle and there was a manure gutter without the metal hardware running between her and the aisle.*

*I squatted down in the gutter, lubricated my right arm, and entered the birth canal with a smooth obstetrical chain in hand. I placed the pre-made loop of chain over the foal's hoof and slid it up over the fetlock. I made another loop and placed that one on the same leg but below the fetlock. My left hand had the other end of the chain outside the mare and I slowly pulled on it to firmly set the loops on the foal's leg.*

*I turned at this point and asked Matt if he was willing to give Dad a hand. Without hesitation, he came over to my side and I handed him the free end of the chain. I placed a chain handle on it and told him to keep pressure on the chain so what I had done would not fall off. He nodded his head in understanding and concentrated on the task. I went back in to locate the other folded back leg and slip on another chain.*

*With both chains in place, it was time to apply traction and draw the limbs out of the canal. This required an orchestration of my free hand pushing the head back into the mare and pulling on one leg, then the other, until they had unfolded. I issued commands to Matt and he followed them exactly. The mare cooperated by remaining on her side and relaxing as I did this.*

*The leg I held unfolded first. I quickly adjusted the handle and gave it to Matt, taking his chain, following it to the other leg, and unfolding that one. Now the foal was in position to be delivered and the mare knew it. She started to push with all of her might. Matt sat in the aisle with his feet pressing up against the gutter wall giving him the mechanical advantage to pull with everything he had. I let Matt and the mare do the work as I witnessed the marvel of my son being like Dad. He pulled and she pushed and the foal finally popped out and took its first breath of air.*

*Matt fell backwards with the biggest look of amazement on his face. The mare motherly nickered and the foal struggled forward towards her noise. This miracle I had seen countless times, but to see it with my son, messy with fetal fluid, smiling broadly, gave me feelings I will never forget.*

*Could it get any better than this? No way!*

# CHAPTER 5

## — *Baby Daddy* —

# CHAPTER 5

Ever since my return from California, I had noticed the development of a respiratory problem whenever I worked in the straw bedded stalls. The invisible dust would fill my nostrils causing the watery mucus to pour out. In time, this dust would start to irritate my throat and then my lungs. I would have difficulty exhaling my air and on some days exhaling would cause a high-pitched squeal.

I lived with this worsening condition until one day I had an extreme bout with some new straw that had arrived on the farm. I slowly and without announcement left the barn I had been working at and walked to my apartment. It was on the second floor and the steps went steeply up the outside of the building. I slowly climbed struggling to get enough air. I walked into the house, calmly found my bedroom and collapsed onto the bed.

I focused hard on breathing. I was starting to pass out. I started to think that I would die. There was no calling anyone. The phone was not in this room and there was no telephone emergency service then. "Inhale slowly and hold it, then exhale," I calmly told myself, but little air came out. I could not empty my lungs. I closed my eyes and relaxed to conserve energy as my body loudly demanded fresh air but I couldn't expel the bad air.

This was asthma and it scared me not just because I thought I might die, but if I lived, I thought my career with horses would be over. About two hours later I felt I could breathe again. I went back outside and found Bill to tell him what had happened. Apparently no one was looking for me. I wonder how long it would have taken before they found my body. That night I went to my parents' for dinner and told them what had happened.

I found a doctor a few days later and had a chest X-ray taken. I had a history of viral pneumonia when I was ten years old, which kept me out of school for two weeks, but now I was wondering if there was a lingering effect.

I was referred to an allergist and then subjected to a hundred skin injections to determine the cause. It was the straw, stupid, yet I was tested for everything under the sun and a serum was developed specifically for me. I was given weekly subcutaneous injections for the next two years to trick my immune system into believing it knew what it was doing. The plan worked and I returned to normal breathing, though when I work at Belmont Park today, 35 years later, where wheat straw is used exclusively, I still pre-medicate with four different drugs to survive the day.

While I almost died laying on my bed at Trotter Farm in 1976, developing and conquering asthma not only proved my determination to work with horses, but it became invaluable on the day of my interview in the acceptance process to veterinary school. It also taught me the one lesson everyone needs to learn. When lemons are served, make some lemonade. And plenty of lemonade was served.

Remembering the first time you did something that had a profound impact on your life is something that never leaves you. The sight, smell, and sounds are seared into memory for no other purpose than to reference the point when a decision was made that affects your life forever. The first time you kissed the girl you end up marrying. The first time you drove the car by yourself. The first foal you pulled out of a mare.

The foaling season starts in January, peaks in April, and fizzles off by June in the United States. Delivery of foals generally occurs in the early morning hours between 3 and 6 am. Detecting those chosen to watch pregnant mares all night and attend these deliveries was easy. Men with unshaved stubble and women with unmade faces, dressed in wrinkled clothes slept in through the previous night often wore hats to cover their messed hair. Walking in a stupor, they joked about everything and yawned between laughs as eyes became distant, then returned to the conversation, and then drifted again. Sleep deprivation comes with the territory and family, friends, and coworkers often give these night creatures the benefit of tolerance until the foaling season is over.

Later in my veterinary career, I would easily pick out the ones up for nights and smile with understanding. They would say, "Doc, I've been up for five nights straight with this mare. You got a shot or something to get this over with?" Hard to know if they wanted relief for them or the horse!

At Trotter Farm I had it lucky. Mrs. Trotter offered Bob, the local police officer that patrolled the town all night, an extra job of being the night watchman of her farm at the same time. He would swing past the farm on his town rounds, stop in the barns where certain mares were due, and when one delivered, make sure all was okay. We were never wakened unless something didn't look right to him, which was fine for all of us with full work days. Most of the time when he returned to the stall with me, the foal would be up and nursing. I didn't care that it was three in the morning and I had a full day's work coming up. Not only did I like this part of the job, I encouraged it.

I always had a set of filet mignons in my refrigerator ready to be cooked thanks to the generosity of the local butcher who had a garden of prized tomatoes. He would exchange his finest meat for bags of straw and horse manure I delivered to him on demand. I was willing to share these mouth-watering steaks with Bob who was willing to let me sleep but would wake me for any problems. Even though I often woke and attended many normal deliveries, Officer Bob and I, both men who were always hungry, would return to my kitchen, cook up a quick steak and laugh and tell stories. I wondered how safe our town was during these early gourmet meals, but I really didn't care. I was setting him up to always call me if a mare needed help. My plan worked flawlessly.

One night, the banging at my back door abruptly woke me into the darkness of a moonless night. It was early spring and the temperature was mild with no wind blowing. I threw on my jeans, shirt, boots, and coat then went to meet Bob at the door. We rapidly descended the stairs and crossed the courtyard as he explained to me that there was something definitely wrong with this mare. He couldn't see the feet of the foal from the birth canal signaling him that there was a delivery problem.

Bob opened the barn door and we entered. The smell of fetal fluid was pungent and was a perfume I would wear many times in my life. I turned the corner and went to the first stall on the left. The mare was laying on her side breathing heavily. Three breaths and then a push with a trumpeting of grunting sounds coming from her flared nostrils and the foal's nose would appear. Then the pushing and grunting sounds would stop and the foal's nose would disappear back inside the mare. She would go back to breathing hard for bit to prepare for the next push and the process would repeat.

I thanked Bob saying, "I think this will be a long night. No time for steak."

Bob wished me good luck and I went back to my apartment to call Dr. Simpson. I then woke up Margaret, the mare's groom, living in the downstairs apartment and asked for her help. It would take forty-five minutes for Dr. Simpson to arrive. That seemed to be a long time I thought, as I returned to the stall.

I needed to do something as the mare continued her cycle of push and rest. The steam lifted off of her sweating body. Her eyes seemed to ask for help as her brow furrowed with worry. I made a decision. I washed her up and then washed my arms, lubricated them with K-Y jelly and entered the birth canal. Margaret stayed on the head.

"This should be easy," I told myself. When a mare delivers, the foal comes out with both front feet first. Between these two long legs is the foal's head. Everything else just follows. I had seen this maybe a dozen times so far and had even had the opportunity to watch Dr. Simpson help deliver a foal. All I had to do was find the legs and pull them out. The rest of the foal should follow.

My arm went slowly inside the warm birth canal while my fingers explored the layers of tissue. The first thing I noticed was the slipperiness of the inner sack. Then I felt the nose. I was surprised when the foal responded to my touch by moving his head. That, as well as the added bulk of my arm, made the mare contract and the pressure on my arm wasn't pleasant but was tolerable. I continued to explore once the contraction ceased.

Both long legs were folded straight back. It reminded me of someone diving into the water from the edge of the pool face first. Most would dive by swinging their arms out in front of them, springing off the edge and entering the water hands first, followed by arms and then head. This is the position of a foal being delivered normally. On occasion, like this foal, someone would keep their hands by their sides, spring off the edge, and land head first into the water. This described the foal's position exactly.

I worked for the whole time it took Dr. Simpson to drive to the farm and enter the barn. I thought I could untangle the legs but all I did was sit nose to nose with the foal. His head popped out rhythmically and was uncovered from his fetal membranes. His blank eyes clearly looked at me each time for a moment until his head disappeared. However, his nose remained next to mine as I continued unsuccessfully to grope at his limbs. My freshman attempt to play veterinarian ended when the real veterinarian entered the barn.

"Hey Geoff, what have we got?" I was both elated that the real vet had arrived and would fix this mess and concerned that he would reprimand me for making the situation worse.

I answered cryptically, "The foal is stuck. I can't find any legs."

Dr. Simpson eyed the scene then turned and asked me directly, "Did you go in her?"

At first I froze knowing I had overstepped my bounds, but then decided to let him know what I had done.

Dr. Simpson, without another word, cleaned up his arms and went inside the mare. In a look I would become familiar with, his eyes stared off into the distance as his mind visualized what his hands and fingers were feeling. Eyes are nothing more than receptors of light energy and that energy is turned into electrical energy that the brain uses to "see." The brain also sees using other sources such as when you walk in the pitch dark from the bedroom to the bathroom. You can see using your memory and your sense of touch as your fingertips gently feel the wall and your feet feel when you cross from carpet to tile. This is what the vet was doing inside the mare.

In a short time, Dr. Simpson pulled his arm out and then without skipping a beat, stood shoulder to shoulder next to me to measure his arm length next to mine. "It looks like your arm is longer than mine Geoff. It's time you finished the job."

Without either one of us batting an eye, Dr. Simpson pulled out the obstetrical chains and began to instruct me on their use. In about three minutes, I became proficient on where to place the chains to avoid damage to the foal as well as the procedure we were to follow in untangling the legs. I was never nervous but I was excited.

I followed his instruction exactly. The chains gave us the leverage needed to manipulate and untangle the limbs ultimately positioning the foal for delivery. It happened quickly. The mare gave a tremendous effort and we pulled the chains down towards her hocks and soon the head, neck, and shoulders with very long chestnut legs appeared. After a moment's rest, another push and grunt from the mare produced the hips and hind limbs down to the hocks. We all stopped and caught our breath.

I had just delivered my first foal and I was floating on a cloud. Dr. Simpson checked the mare and the foal, told me I had done a great job, then left along with Margaret. I stayed for a while marveling as the hair coat on the foal dried. He struggled to get up and nurse and with a little help from his mother he did. I realized that my path with horses was set and there was no turning back. Never had I felt so sure about anything. With that, I went back to my bed and took a two-hour nap before the day's work.

I did not return to the mare until nearly 10 am in the morning. Others were there to clean the stall and take care of the mare and foal. As I approached the barn I knew something was wrong. Dr. Simpson was there along with Mrs. Trotter in the barn courtyard. Margaret was walking the mare in a circle within the yard allowing the foal to follow. The two looked gravely at the foal. That is when I noticed the dropped pasterns allowing the fetlocks to touch the ground. In addition, the legs from the hocks and knees down were twisted and week. As the foal moved, the limbs swayed sideways. He did not want to move by himself and another groom was pushing him along from behind.

I had arrived from another barn and needed to deliver something so I went around the corner of the barn dropping off the item. I came back around the corner suddenly into the courtyard. The mare and foal looked up at me. What happened next still astonishes me.

The foal saw me, left his mother's side, and walked on his own crossing the full diameter of the courtyard to me. Both Mrs. Trotter and Dr. Simpson had never seen anything like that before. With her hands on her hips and her mouth gaping, Mrs. Trotter attempted to pull herself together. With a slight smile and what some would call a perturbed look, she announced, "Geoff, go out of sight again and let the foal rejoin his mother."

She never really said that I was to come back. It was silly of her to think that a newborn foal could possibly be attached to me. Mrs. Trotter's dignity instructed her to brush the incident aside, but her inner child was allowed to escape that morning which allowed me to test the theory.

Did the foal recognize me and did it place more importance on me than anyone else there including his mother? I waited for a minute sneaking a peak around the corner of the barn. When the mare and foal had made a turn and a half around the grass and dirt square courtyard and the pair was directly across and 20 yards away, I came around into the opposite corner. The foal saw me and again left his mother walking on his own weak limbs the full distance across the grass into my arms.

Everyone came over with looks of amazement. The mare nickered and poked her head in to break things up. I guided the foal back to the nursing position and he gladly guzzled. Mrs. Trotter declared her amazement saying she had never seen such an event. She seemed almost proud for a moment, then dismissed the fuss and headed back to the barn ordering Margaret to bring the mare and foal back into the stall.

Dr. Simpson came up to me and told me that I had imprinted myself on the foal when we were nose to nose for the first hour of its life. Through seemingly blank eyes, the foal had seen me as his mother. More astonishingly, he saw me at a distance and recognized me. I was moved beyond words and my feelings were loud inside my body. This is where I wanted to be. Horses were my life and nothing would change this. The connection between me, the mare, and this foal became the very foundation of my existence as a horseman on which everything else in my life has been built upon. My path to becoming a veterinarian was set, but I still was not aware of this as a possibility in my life.

# POP!

*The barrel racehorse fired out of the gate carrying her rider towards the first barrel. Her body leaned at a 45° angle as the barrel rocked in her wind. The rider looked at the next barrel and the horse understood. She dug in with everything she had. Reaching the second barrel she started braking and turning.*

POP! *The horse immediately fell and slid into the wall of the arena of the State Fair Grounds in Syracuse, New York. The rider was safe and immediately examined his mare, the horse of more concern than himself. She stood up and was non-weight bearing on her left foreleg. The owner lived several hours away and quickly asked local people which vet to call. My name was chosen. I received the call, listened carefully to his story, and told him that I was on my way. Quickly gathering my equipment and supplies for a broken leg, I jumped into my truck and headed north on Interstate 81 for 45 minutes.*

*The State Fairgrounds is an asphalt parking lot with a big arena in the center. Surrounding outbuildings included stalls for the visiting horses. There is no grass except for islands about 10 feet long and 4 feet wide scattered in the parking lot. I found the horse and owner in a barn near the parking lot and began my exam. The pastern was swelling and my fingers felt the crepitus as the broken pieces of pastern bone crunched within the limb.*

*"Good news!" I said with a positive tone. "The skin is not broken so your horse has a good chance for this to heal without complications."*

*The owner appeared to be a man unshakable to most things, but for this horse, he had assumed I would perform euthanasia. With his eyes blinking, he stammered, "Heal? You mean you can help her?"*

*I replied, "This is a clean wound with no dirt in the broken bones. I can cast this leg. She will never race again, but she will certainly live a good and pain free life."*

*"You mean I could breed her and have a foal?"*

*My answer of "Yup" brought a spark back to him and the mare sensed it.*

*"I need a farrier here now and I need to move some vehicles away from that island. You ready?"*

*I placed a catheter into her left jugular and administered some sedative and painkiller. Then I instructed the owner to move his pick up to a position that I pointed out. The farrier arrived and I instructed him to make a heart bar shoe for the good front limb. I also asked him to place a 3/16th inch bit in his drill and hunted for some baling wire and some warm water.*

*I placed everything I needed in the bed of the pickup then slowly led the mare out toward the island of grass. Anesthetizing this horse and having it land within a small patch of grass was like landing a 747 airliner on a backyard landing strip. She wobbled as the drugs kicked in. I pushed and tugged her head adjusting her gentle fall perfectly in the middle of the grass strip with her legs toward the pickup and her back facing the large utility pole at the end of the island. It was a long shot that she would land perfectly, but the odds could not outdo my will for this to happen.*

*The farrier then went to work. He removed both front shoes and trimmed the hoof on the broken leg. He handed me the drill and I drilled a hole through the toe of the hoof. He then continued to work on making the shoe and applying it to the good leg.*

*While he worked, I ran the one-inch thick tow rope I had brought under the mare's body around the girth and attached the ends to the utility pole. I cut and threaded the baling wire through the hoof hole and made it into a loop. Attaching one hook from my come-along winch to the loop, I attached the other end of the come-along to the truck's bumper. I winched up the slack and then applied traction to the leg. The limb was about one foot off the ground and parallel to it. There was a direct line from the bumper, along the winch cable, through the toe, up the leg, through the rope, and onto the utility pole. This could not go any better.*

*I applied the casting material incorporating a block of wood under the heel and a cutting wire to cut off the cast without injuring the leg. The fiberglass hardened within minutes. I released the traction and cut the ends of the wire flush then removed the rope. The farrier was done with his work. We cleared the area and in another few minutes, as if she knew we were done, the mare started to wake. In five minutes, she was standing. We all looked on in amazement as she placed full weight on the broken leg and slowly walked back to the stall. She was hungry and told us so. Thirty minutes later, she stood quietly in the stall munching on hay with full weight on her injured leg.*

*I never saw the man or his mare again, but for many years in the spring he sent me a photo of his mare with that year's newborn foal at her side along with a note of thanks.*

# CHAPTER 6

*— Dyslexia —*

# CHAPTER 6

Now firmly placed on a career path with a future of becoming the farm manager of Trotter Farm, I started to reflect on my life. I wondered why I was so poor at school. I didn't feel stupid and I often felt I was a lot smarter than most of my former classmates. I could learn things easily, but the grades weren't there to prove it. Add to this my unsuccessful attempts at college and doubt crept into my thoughts. The responsibility of a farm manager required not only hard work, but also clear thought. I wondered if I would be successful in my newly found career or if my lack of ability in school would catch up with me.

I loved horses, but details never lingered long in my mind. Lineages of horses were impossible to recreate correctly thus putting me at a disadvantage in the breeding aspect of the industry. On the flip side, I became very successful when working with all the horses. As if I could read their minds, I connected with all the mares that would come to the farm for breeding or foaling.

I couldn't focus much on my inadequacies though because we were in the middle of foaling season and there was not much time to think. When I did unexpectedly get a moment off one afternoon, I decided to visit my parents who were living 20 minutes away. Dad was still at work in Manhattan so Mom and I took advantage of the brilliant spring day to sit in lawn chairs outside the house. This right to spring is often done on days when the temperature gets above 50 degrees. We were wearing coats to stay warm as we sat eating a tomato and lettuce sandwich with garlic salt and mayonnaise in our attempt to fool ourselves into thinking it was summer.

With our late lunch gone we sat quietly enjoying the above freezing temperatures. My mind swirled as it has always done since childhood. A random thought came up and stayed. The thought was about me going to the vocational school while I was still in high school to take remedial reading courses. This was along with the special classes I was placed in after the regular school classes and in summer school. I was given a story to read followed by a series of questions to test our comprehension of the story. The instructor then "taught" me to read by forcing me to place my finger under the first word of the first sentence. He then instructed me to draw my finger under the line moving it from left to right. My eyes were to follow reading the words one at a time until I reached the end of the line. At this point my finger was to move to the next line down taking my eyes with it so I would begin to read the next line. I was to repeat this process until all the lines were read.

My eyes would do as they were told for at most two lines after which they went wherever they wanted to go. Usually they went to the opposite side of the page of where my finger went. The eyes would move from right to left crossing the path the finger was making as it went from left to right.

As I progressed I would be moved up a scale of difficulty that was identified by the color of the books. I never made it past the halfway point and I became discouraged. It was this feeling that had risen above my swirling thoughts that afternoon with Mom. I decided to ask her about it.

"Mom, what were all those tests I took when I was in high school?"

"What tests?" she asked.

"You remember, after school and at the vocational school where they made me read all those stupid little books."

What she said next stunned me. "Oh those tests! Well, they said something like you had difficulty reading. I think they said you read from right to left instead of left to right."

For the first time in my life, someone told me why I couldn't read! After a poor high school record and three attempts at college, now I knew. "Mom! That's called dyslexia!"

"Really," she said as she took a sip of ice tea. "What's dyslexia?"

I said in disbelief, "It's when someone reads backwards."

The educators never thought it was important to explain to my parents or me what they had discovered about me. Maybe it was because they knew little about this newly discovered syndrome. Maybe it was because not telling us was the way educators were taught to treat non-conforming students. I will never know why they never told us but my distrust of the education system started that day. Another thing that started that very moment was my determination to learn how to read.

There is an expression that says, "When the student is ready, the teacher will appear." My teacher appeared on TV with an advertisement for the Evelyn Wood Speed Reading course with a free introductory seminar at the Mt. Kisco Holiday Inn the following week. I went and was amazed at what was presented. I signed up and bought the training books but I never went to any of the classes. I just read their material and began to understand how my brain worked.

The best way to explain how I read is to imagine an empty room inside my head. As I read the words on the page, the words enter into the empty room and swirl around in a blur. In a moment, they settle down onto the floor of the room. They can be upside down or on end as well as right side up. Now I take the words and arrange them into a structure using the rules for sentence syntax. In a moment, the words start to come into focus and the meaning of the sentence becomes evident. The sentence is now allowed to leave the room and more words are then allowed to enter. The process repeats itself until what I'm reading is finished.

This is a very slow process. In the past everyone was telling me how to read fast, I skipped over words and sentences in an effort to keep up. If I slowed down and did the process my way, I was left behind. I can't remember what it was about the Evelyn Wood Speed Reading process that clicked with me. Between the course and just knowing that I read differently, not incorrectly, gave my self-confidence the boost it needed for me to advance. I felt strong and I started to experiment on reading techniques that worked for me.

I found a book in my dad's library called *Sun Up* by Will James. A story about a cowboy's life a hundred years ago, I became enraptured with his stories. From his experience with horses, I became a better horseman as well as a better reader. Over the next year I worked on the process of changing everything I had been taught about reading. I discovered the slowest part was putting the puzzle together. I started with license plates.

As I drove I would look at the plate on the car in front of me and allow the numbers and letters to float into my room. I used my eyes like a shutter on a camera. I briefly closed my eyes then rapidly opened and closed them like a camera's shutter taking in the plate numbers. Yes, I know, I was driving at the time and maybe this wasn't the safest thing to do but the process didn't take long. It was short but each step had to occur in order for me to "see" the plate. As I saw the letters and numbers swirl into my room, I quickly learned to arrange what I saw. When done, I would open my eyes and compare my answer to the plate in front of me.

Once I learned to trust the process, my accuracy rose. Once my accuracy neared 100% I graduated myself from license plates to whole exit signs. The secret was to take in the whole text as an image rather than word by word. As I increased my confidence, I started to read more books and magazines.

Over the next 18 months I gradually improved to where I thought I could try school again. I also realized that I was not stupid or slow. I just think differently and my conviction was correct and fully justified. I also realized that this might have been a blessing. It is because of this dyslexia that I ended up in a career I never dreamed I would be in. Only a few more hurdles to clear before becoming a vet. But learning to read probably was the biggest.

# TOM AND ROCKETS – THE SAGA

*"Doc, This is Tom. Can you come quick? Rockets' in trouble!"*

*Usually this is where the story begins, but this is more than a story. It is a saga.*

*Tom's Quarter Horse, Rockets, had been a patient of mine for years. He is what a vet would call a routine horse. No emergencies ever occurred and the usual visit was for preventive things. Minor scrapes or a worried eye were usually addressed simply and with one visit. "In trouble" were words I had never heard from Tom.*

*In fact, the "trouble" had been mostly with Tom as he and his wife went through difficult times. They were now divorced. Solace was found by preparing Rockets for this day. It had been a dream of Tom's to ride his horse from upstate New York down to Texas, into Mexico, and through Central America into South America along the Pan American Highway. After the divorce, he scheduled his early retirement from his job at Cornell and began to sell off everything he owned. Today, all he had was on his and Rockets' back.*

*The day was wet. A spring rain soaked the leaves and created a double rain where you could be hit with a soft raindrop or a heavier one of accumulated drops on a leaf. This of course caused a drenched feeling where no part of land remained dry. It was this day that Tom had scheduled to leave for the southern* hemisphere. I would have slept in and waited for dry weather, but Tom was excited. Nothing was going to stop him.

As he rode Rockets down the hill toward the main road, I'm sure the boy inside of him was leaping around, but he was the type that showed little emotion on the outside. Down the road the lazy, unemotional pair drew closer to the first of many forks in the road.

The excitement he was trying to suppress leaked into Rockets' body. Ahead on the main road, before the first turn south was a construction crew laying a long and large pale green pipe. Rockets' eyes grew large. Nothing in his training with Tom had prepared him for this. Nervously he placed his hooves in directions that Tom had not planned. Tom stopped and calmed his horse aware he was losing his connection. He then dismounted and once he felt he had Rockets' attention, he assured him it would be okay and if he just followed the leader, they could both walk past the big mean yellow monsters with the long green snake.

"Nope!" said Rockets as he refused to follow.

Tom, looking for an alternative, saw it in a railroad track running parallel to the road. Acting on his impromptu plan, he led Rockets back to the railroad grade and turned north where he could detour around the construction. All was going well but in about 100 feet at eye level, an invisible bridge appeared. It spanned about 40 feet and was made of railroad ties that were about 12 inches wide and spaced about 10 inches apart. "Only 40 ties to cross. No big deal. Rockets would surely follow," Tom thought. "He's my friend and he trusts me."

Ten feet across the bridge, Rockets' hoof slipped on the rain soaked timber and his left foreleg fell between the ties. His body thudded on the ties and the animal started to panic. Tom, trying not to fall himself, calmed his horse but deep inside he panicked too. He grabbed his phone and dialed me. This is when he said, "Doc, this is Tom. Can you come quick? Rockets' in trouble!"

Off in the distance, an approaching northbound train blew its' whistle.

I felt helpless as I heard Tom's words. I was an hour away with a lot of unpredictable traffic in between us.

I advised him to get someone else to attend. His story of Rockets falling through a railroad bridge seemed beyond the scope of a veterinarian. However, I had learned early in my career that a veterinarian does not attend to the animals needs, but they attend to the needs of the animal's owner through their animal. So I said, "Get some help now and I will be there as fast as I can."

I called the New York State Troopers and asked for an escort. I worried that the snarls of traffic between the interstate and the horse would add time I did not have. Tom had painted a grim picture, but not grim enough to encourage the police to help. I was on my own.

*Luckily Tom was not. You could see Rockets and Tom from the main road. Attention grew and people gathered. Whenever people see something not fitting the pattern of normalcy, like seeing a person with three eyes, it forces them to come and stare. Usually the crowd becomes mesmerized into inaction, but on occasion, if the circumstances are right, the people will galvanize together and help. That is what this crowd did as the northbound coal train approached.*

*One nameless man turned towards the sound and ran as fast as he could waving his coat. The engineer said later that due to the warm weather, his cars loaded with coal for the heating plant were empty. He was heading north to the salt mines by the lake to pick up a load of salt. Had he been loaded, he never would have been able to stop in time. The running man had taken good action at the right time and Rockets received a break.*

*Another man seeing the train had stopped realized that this horse had to be extracted now. He also saw the pipe laying construction crew along the main road and went to plead with the foreman. He did well because shortly there was a crane hovering above the horse. By now the University vets had arrived to sedate Rockets and give painkiller. The crowd brought their hands and strength together and passed straps under Rockets. Soon he was high above the tracks and being swung to safety.*

*To everyone's amazement, especially Tom's, Rockets slowly started to walk. He was bruised and cut in many areas. The vet* offered to help but Tom said, "No thank you. My vet will be here any minute." He walked Rockets back to his barn and made him comfortable.

I had missed all the action but I was soon to work attending to the cuts and abrasions. It took three hours. During this time as Tom replayed what had happened, I saw the shock he was going through. This is where the real work of a veterinarian starts. Suturing a gaping cut is easy. Mending an owner's mind filled with guilt, doubt, and fear is harder. Maybe I only needed an hour or so to actually care for the horse, but Tom needed the full three hours I spent there that day.

As Rockets munched on hay, Tom made some coffee, then said, "Geoff, I think I won't go on this trip." I asked why. He recited his list of reasons formulated in his head that day.

I said, "Tom, you have been no less traumatized by this than Rockets. You need time to heal. I will come back every day until I know both of you are doing better." I went on to say, "These minor wounds will be fine to move on in about two weeks. You have two weeks to work things out. Don't let fear stop you from living your dream. You need to face fear and realize that it is only your perception and right now you feel guilty for leading Rockets over that bridge. Get over it cause he already has!"

With that we paused and looked at his horse lazily munching on the pile of hay. He was living in the moment. He did not show any signs of resentment. He looked content and Tom gave a brief smile.

It took two weeks for all the wounds to heal. It took a month for Tom's wounds to heal. On a quiet late summer morning, they both left town never to return.

Tom never realized his dream of following the Pan American Highway across Central America into South America. At the Rio Grand bridge between the US and Mexico border, the authorities said he was not allowed to ride the horse across the bridge. He could trailer it, but this was not his dream. He made a fuss and soon the Laredo newspaper caught wind of it. Tom sent me the front page with a large picture of him and Rockets above the fold that told their story. A ground swell of support for them started. A woman came forward and offered Tom and Rockets a place to stay until the crossing became resolved.

The letter Tom wrote to me had me choking with tears of joy. The woman who offered him shelter became his soul mate and they had decided to marry.

I lost track of Tom and Rockets after that, but for all I know, Tom is happily married living in Texas.

Remember this: For every dream you have, follow it no matter what obstacle gets in your path. Look at adversity as an opportunity. Never let fear be an excuse for not taking action.

# CHAPTER 7

## — *Barn Girl* —

# CHAPTER 7

One of my new duties at Trotter Farm was learning to break yearlings for riding. Back then the term "breaking" did not have a stigma attached to it as it does today. What we did was organized and tailored to each individual horse we trained. Most breakings were uneventful and we never used force. It is exactly what the "natural horsemen" use today.

We worked in teams and I was teamed with Sunny. I became the ground man introducing the young horse to the bit and the saddle and the pressure of the girth. It became my laboratory for discovering how to first listen to the horse and then to be understood. It is where I developed two-way communication with horses as a way to establish trust. Some horses were quicker than others but we always took our time proving patience was quicker than the quick beating-and-demand method.

The first step in breaking horses at the farm always started right after birth. Every foal was haltered on day one and taught leadership. Leading the foal ahead of the mare rather than allowing it to follow the mare easily teaches confidence. This one procedure alone, if done by every horse owner with a newborn foal, would reduce ill-mannered horses tremendously.

When the foal entered the spring of their second year, every foal was not only tractable; they were usually willing to learn new things. Having the young horse now accept a halter with a Chifney bit attached was usually easy. They soon would have a bridle and bit comfortably in the mouth. Next I would place a jockey's exercise saddle on the back. I called the small saddle a postage stamp. It weighed maybe two pounds without the girth. This was placed on the back then off the back then back again until the two year old understood the new idea.

The most important part of training a horse is to know when to stop. Learning one little lesson may have taken only five minutes, but then it was time to stop, congratulate, and wait a day before teaching another lesson. Breaking down the process into many small steps is how I describe "breaking" a horse but it is how a horse learns, through assurance and repetition. It is the same way humans learn when you get right down to it.

The next step was to attach the saddle to the horse using a girth. Tightening the girth often sent a few youngsters into a tizzy but it was short lived and with little conviction on the part of the horse. We always broke the horse in a 12-foot by 12-foot stall with a 20-foot high ceiling. I stood in the center of the stall and the horse had a halter on and a lead rope attached. I stuck the free end deep into my right front pocket. Now I still had access to control the horse only a short distance from my right hand yet both of my hands were free to work with the horse. I placed the saddle on the horse and had him take a turn around the stall. Next I attached the girth and snugged it up tight enough to keep the saddle in place but not so tight to be uncomfortable. We would take another turn or two around the stall.

I continued this process slowly over a few days depending on the acceptance by the yearling. At some point, the girth became tight enough to carry the weight of a rider. This is where Sunny came into the picture. In the stall I stood quietly in the center with the haltered horse in hand. Sunny stood quietly next to me. She was as small as a jockey. She would hold onto the saddle using her left hand on the front of it and her right hand on the back of it. She would stand on her right leg while she bent her left leg back 90 degrees at the knee.

With my left hand holding the halter, my right arm would be down at my side with my right hand cupped around Sunny's bent left lower leg just above her ankle. We counted to three. I lifted her straight up and she would land as light as a feather with her stomach on the saddle. We called this "bellying the horse." At the same time, I asked the horse to move forward to place the horse's energy in any direction other than straight up. Almost without exception this was done without incident. Occasionally the horse would hop a little but this was kept under control and the student would easily settle down.

The final step of my job was setting the rider on top of the horse with both legs on each side of the horse. The sequence was belly the horse, turn once in the stall then off; belly, turn once, then off. Then it was rider up, turn once, then off. I gave a pat on the neck and it was on to the next horse.

The day soon came when the horse had to be ridden in the stall without me. Sunny would teach the horse to move forward within the stall. She would turn the horse using the bit to go the other way in the stall. Finally, when the lessons were learned and the horse was ready, I would open the gate and Sunny would ride the horse out of the stall, turn left, and ride the horse for the first time down the shed row. Again most horses did this well but on occasion, some spirited horses would become a handful as they jumped up or went sideways as they experienced their freedom outside the stall but now with a lump of human on their back.

Sunny and I made a good team and I learned a lot from her years of doing this. I was looking forward to repeating the process with the next batch of horses that needed breaking. This was scheduled for May.

I heard that a new girl was starting over at the pony barn. I considered it part of my job to introduce myself to any new help. Usually I would just come across the new employee as I did my job, but word had gotten out quickly on the farm that she was good looking. I decided that I soon had business to do at the pony barn knowing I'd run into her.

She had just dipped two pails of water into the old-fashioned bathtub used as a stock tank filled with drinking water. She turned around to walk toward where I had just entered the pony yard. Carrying two full buckets of water is difficult enough without the curves of a woman's hips interfering. With each step she took the buckets moved beyond their ability to contain the water. Her pant legs were wet with splashed water and her face beaded with sweat. Still, her clear green eyes sparkled. Long brown hair was parted in the middle and swept back to each side tied into a ponytail that swayed as she walked. Her eyes met mine and she smiled. Time stopped – for me at least.

"Hi. I'm Geoff, the assistant farm manager. I mostly work at the training barn but I had heard there was a new person over here so I came over to introduce myself." At least that's what I had planned to say. I can't remember what actually came out of my mouth. I was like a zombie mumbling sounds that must have been incoherent to any linguist. I remember she said her name was Kathy. I quickly turned and left.

I found more reasons to "run into her" as my mornings filled with excitement of the possibility of seeing Kathy again. I hadn't realized the reason for the farm hiring her was to help break the new batch of horses. When she showed up at the training barn early in June, I was crazy with excitement because now I'd see her a great deal. When I found I would be teamed up with her instead of Sunny, I had mixed emotions. I loved working with the young horses and Sunny and I did it well. I was excited to be with Kathy but her abilities as a horseman were unknown to me.

That worry was short lived as we started working together going through the process of bellying and backing the young horses. We had fun together and I felt comfortable for the first time with a girl. I decided to ask her out and we went to Friendly's Restaurant for dinner. It was our first date and underneath the table we held hands. I was being hooked like a lazy catfish on a warm summer day, but I didn't mind one bit.

Sometimes we think we are in control of life but later find out we were just along for the ride. About a year before Kathy had met me she was at a party with a boyfriend she'd had since high school. The group decided to break out the Ouija board, dim the lights, light some candles, and ask the board questions to get whatever mysterious answers that were waiting from 'beyond.' Everyone there assumed that Kathy was going to be with her boyfriend forever so they asked the board who she was going to marry. It was their test to see if the board really worked and could read the future.

The board piece had four small "legs." On the bottom of each leg was a thick piece of felt allowing it to effortlessly move on the board's surface. It was big enough to allow six people to place their fingertips on top. This allowed the "energy" of the spirits to travel through the fingertips causing the piece to move. As it did, the pointer on it would pass over letters allowing the spirits to spell messages.

The stand where people placed their fingers now started to move across the board. The pointer stopped at the first letter - G. It moved again and again spelling G-E-O-F-F. Most people didn't even know that it was the old English spelling of Jeff and passed it off as a fluke. Even Kathy had not remembered that night until she called a friend to tell her about the date with the new boy she had met. From that point on, Kathy knew she would be marrying me. She never told me and I was left to my own devices to figure this out. Thankfully, it didn't take me long.

Kathy and I had finished our work on a horse located in the first stall on the backside of the barn just past the middle of the barn break. She was sitting on top of the horse and I was turning her a few times around in the stall. All was going well and it was time for Kathy to ride the big black filly out of the stall into the shed row. I removed the lead and she did another turn around me in the stall. As they passed the gate, I stepped forward, opened the gate all the way, and walked out of the stall and around the corner into the middle break.

I waited as Kathy made one more revolution before leading the filly out. The horse, however, had other plans. The filly rose on her hind legs and in a fully erect posture, walked out of the stall like a human, turned left and remaining on her hind legs, walked down the shed row past the middle break. My mouth became dry as I held my breath waiting for the inevitable disaster to occur. I could imagine Kathy falling to the earth in a broken heap as the horse ran off. Instead, I only saw Kathy riding perfectly balanced laughing at the ridiculousness of the filly's behavior. She dug her heels into the horse and shouted "Git going!" which sent the filly back on all four legs trotting nicely in the direction Kathy wanted to go.

I was amazed (and relieved!) then made up my mind right there that I was going to marry Kathy. In September, 1976, after three months of knowing her, I proposed. While she didn't say "yes," she also didn't say "no." She knew her answer already but I guess she just wanted to be sure I was the right G-E-O-F-F.

# IS MY HORSE PREGNANT?

*The looks on their faces were drawn and serious. I was nervous, as it was my first year on the job as a veterinarian.*

*I worked for a rural general practice where I saw mostly cows and small animals. My boss could work on horses but was glad to hire someone showing interest in them so he could concentrate on the cows of the upstate New York hills where he was born and raised.*

*Daryl and Betsy are a husband and wife that enjoyed each other's company and brought an air of perfection to everything they did. They were always clean and so were their Quarter Horses and the barn. "Neat" would be their description I would apply followed with "serious." They were proud of their Swedish roots and reminded me of it often.*

*Today was not my first visit. I had done enough things right on their farm to earn their suspicious trust but I was far from absolutely proving myself to them. Today they wanted my opinion of several things including a pregnancy exam. I started in on the list and the items were simple and straightforward.*

*"I want you to check if this horse is pregnant," Daryl said is a stern and authoritative voice as we approached the final item on his list. He had been a magistrate in the past and was used to saying things once and getting the correct results immediately. He also proudly owned a Thompson sub-machine gun and all I could*

think of was he was a lawman from the old whiskey running days and he took no prisoners.

Betsy slipped a halter and lead rope on the horse and I followed her into the stall. My brain was filled with images of how this tall "Abe Lincoln" looking man with a trimmed black beard peppered with gray hairs continued to size me up. His questioning eyes challenged me constantly and he had every right to do this. I was fresh out of vet school and my fingertips had little experience in pregnancy detection. Fancy technology did not exist. We were just grateful for plastic sleeves and the word ultrasound was not even on the horizon.

Let's not let Betsy off the hook on this scrutiny of me. While her piercing blue Scandinavian eyes, full blond hair, and tight fitting jeans sculpted her body and reminded me of pictures I had seen in magazines in my pre-marriage days, her look was no less stern than Daryl's when it came to their horses.

Seriousness settled in as I started to position myself behind the horse and I applied copious amounts of lubricant to the sleeve on my arm. My young vet mind dove deep into my training. My thoughts did a dry run: Slowly enter one finger, then two, then my whole hand into the horse's rectum. Stand to one side in case the horse decided to kick. Evacuate the manure from the rectum then re-lube. Work my way into the rectum slowly and dip my curved fingers down towards the pelvis and "hook" the uterus. Work my hand both to the left and to the right and feel for uterine *tone and any large lumps. At this point in my thinking, my brain stopped. Something wasn't right.*

*I had my sleeve on and the lube was dripping off it, but that was as far as I had gotten. I turned to the couple and asked the breeding date. It was the fall and this horse should be anywhere from 3 to 9 months pregnant. Why were they asking me to check this mare now when the size of the foal would be very large and they should have had the mare confirmed pregnant months ago? Daryl's response was annoying. "You tell me Doc."*

*I lifted the tail and aimed my forefinger towards the anus. I froze. One hole! I stopped and looked up at the two who had twitching corners on their lips. "What the heck," I exclaimed!*

*Darryl and Betsy started to uncontrollably laugh as they pranced around their quiet-as-a-mouse stallion saying that they had got their new young vet to do a rectal on their stallion to see if he was pregnant.*

*I protested, "I never went in! I did NOT do a rectal on a stallion for pregnancy!"*

*This only fueled their fire and they told this story to anyone who would listen for the next few years.*

*I went home mad and upset, but I also went home knowing I would be their vet forever. And I was.*

# CHAPTER 8
## — *A Blind Horse Guides Me* —

# CHAPTER 8

I was absorbing mountains of information about the medical care of horses as I went about doing my job on the farm. Each day brought something new and almost all of it was good. I was now in charge of recording all preventive care for every horse. In addition, I was in charge of all treatments.

This promotion in my mind was the expression of confidence I needed from Walt. Our relationship was tenuous since the day he overheard me say something terrible about him. The words from my mouth were still lingering in the air when he appeared from around the corner of the barn. He looked straight into my eyes, then turned and walked away. I regretted it immediately.

To my knowledge, I had never hurt anyone with my words. Maybe I was lucky or maybe I'll just never know of the damage I may have done. My parents and grandparents never used spiteful words, but on that day in the long training barn, I had something to say about Walt and it was destructive. Of course it was said as a joke, but there was no laughter as I stared into Walt's face.

To this day I never say anything about someone unless I am willing to say it in front of them. I also learned something else from this event. When you do something wrong, you must apologize no matter how hard it is for you to do so. This is what I did with Walt. Weeks later, when I'd decided that I just had to tell him how very sorry I was, he found my apology to be sincere and my actions around him to be noble. Walt forgave me and began to trust me by giving me more responsibilities on the farm.

This went well until the day he said to me, "Grab that eye ointment and start treating that filly's eye in the small barn." I knew that the two-year-old black filly had injured her right eye. There were tears streaming down her face from the half-shut eye.

I immediately went back to the training barn and in the medicine cabinet I found several partially squeezed tubes of eye ointment. Each had very small print identifying their ingredients. The words were big and meant nothing to me. I grabbed the least dirty tube with the most ointment in it and returned to the filly's stall. Medicating that eye three to four times a day became my reason for working the next few days. She was calm as I parted her lids and squeezed the tube ejecting an inch or more of gray gel across the clear part of her eye. The problem was, though, that the eye was not getting better. The clear part was now gray and opaque. She still squinted her eye and the tears still flowed. I reported this to Walt who immediately accused me of not treating the eye.

I was in shock that he thought I was incompetent or at worse, too lazy to attend to this horse properly. I became unsure of my abilities as the words of my mentor rang in my ears. My stomach churned as he said that he was calling the vet.

Later that afternoon Dr. Simpson arrived and quickly entered the barn using the efficiency of a man fitting us into his busy schedule. The barn was dark enough for his exam and he brought his ophthalmoscope up to the eye. In five seconds, he dropped his arm, swung around to Walt, and asked firmly, "What have you been treating this eye with?"

Caught off guard, Walt stuttered then said, "With eye ointment."

"Let me see it," Dr. Simpson barked. The words on the tube had meaning to the educated man. He dropped his shoulders then said, "This medicine is harming the eye, not helping it. This ingredient allows the infection to become worse."

While Dr. Simpson was disappointed, Walt looked like he had been beaten. Not only had he shown a weakness in his ability as a trainer, he knew he had been wrong in accusing me of incompetence. Although he spoke infrequently to me over the next few weeks, he did his best to show me he was sorry. For me it wasn't about receiving an apology. It was about being asked to do something that was wrong and not knowing any better. I became angry with myself and decided to ask Dr. Simpson about it the next chance that I had.

An eye specialist along with Dr. Simpson attended to the treatment of this filly. It included surgery at his hospital and the installation of a tube under the skin of her eye for easier treatment on the hourly schedule. Even with this advanced and aggressive treatment, the mare lost her eye. I cornered Dr. Simpson alone soon after and, mostly from guilt, asked him how I could have done something so stupid.

He looked at me squarely and said, "Why don't you become a vet?"

Laughing out loud, I asked if he was kidding.

He smiled and said, "Why not? You are good with horses and are a hard worker."

Of all things, I said next, "How would I be able to pay for that?"

It's funny how we easily and immediately start to list the reasons why we can't or shouldn't do something rather than saying, "Why not?"

Dr. Simpson recognized my defense and said, "Don't worry about the cost. Just go do it."

I returned home after work and laid out the idea to Kathy. She, without hesitation, gave her fullest support saying, "You were meant to be more than just a manager for this farm."

My mind raced into swirling thoughts that made no sense. I couldn't read, had dropped out of college (three times!), and didn't have any money. I could never be a doctor, I thought. I'm not smart enough, I'm lazy, and I'm scared – that was the real truth of it. What if I tried and failed? I didn't think I could live a life without horses.

Dr. Simpson and Kathy, however, both said I could do it. It was that night when the clarity of vision formed in my mind. Two of the most trusted people in my life had said to me on the same day, "Geoff, you can do it." Yes, I was scared of failure, but what if I succeeded? What if?

## A RARE FOALING DISASTER

*Except for one or two foal deliveries, just about every story about them could start with, "It was a dark and stormy night…." So it was on this night as I carefully drove my vet truck to Janet's Thoroughbred breeding farm.*

*Her call had a sense of urgency from an otherwise unflappable and jolly young woman who always smiled and worked very hard. I visited her farm about every other day during the breeding season and like so many other women during the sleepless time of foaling several mares, her face showed the toll of fatigue.*

*"Got a bad one Doc," she said over the phone.*

*I threw my clothes on and left the warm house and entered the pitch-black cold. Forty-five minutes later I was looking down at a mare lying on her left side with half of her body lying outside the stall door in the aisle. Her dead foal had already been removed. She was breathing rapidly and her heart rate was elevated. A quick look gave the obvious diagnosis of shock caused by a prolapsed uterus. Lying on the barn floor by her tail, the familiar texture of the uterus' exposed lining was clearly seen in the dim barn light.*

*I attended quickly to her state of shock. In an effort to stabilize her, I emptied the truck of everything I could think of to help. I waited for several bags of fluids to course through her system and for the heart to respond. My mind raced for the solution to her dilemma and wondered why she seemed more affected by it than I would expect.*

*A prolapse of the uterus occurs during the birth event when the mare not only pushes out the foal and placenta, but the uterus as well. It is more common in the cow and I had successfully replaced several of them in my first year as a vet when I worked in a dairy practice. However, a prolapse was a rare event in a mare.*

*With my mind clearly set in a plan of action, I wrapped the tail of the mare, still laying on her side, and tied it out of the way. I set to washing the dirt and straw from the exposed uterus as well as the back of the horse. In the middle of this, I was able to see under the uterus and my heart stopped. I froze in place with dread washing over me.*

*Janet saw my reaction and asked, "What's wrong Geoff?"*

*I lifted the uterus fully out of the way blinking in disbelief as I identified the intestines of the mare lying underneath. The mare was all but dead and nothing more could be done. I looked up at Janet's distraught and drawn face as I left to get the euthanasia solution and put the mare to sleep.*

*Ninety out of 100 deliveries of foals go without a hitch. Nine out of ninety get stuck a little and need some help. This delivery was the one in 100 that was a complete disaster and no amount of training or knowledge would have helped her. Janet was as experienced as they come but she missed this one. There was nothing she could have done either.*

*These are times when I wished for just a touch of that God-like quality I used to think vets possessed. Some magic that could repair the un-repairable, stop time turning, and have everything turn out okay. However all you can do is to understand that this is just the way of nature and still do your best for every animal that needs help.*

# CHAPTER 9

*— A Soul Speaks Volumes —*

# Chapter 9

In the 1970's, I thought veterinarians were right up there with God as far as miracle workers - at least they must sit on his board of directors. They could listen to non-speaking animals and tell what was wrong. They had knowledge that was beyond mere mortal man in my opinion and I was both mystified and intrigued. I was just a stall cleaner turned horse farm manager learning as I went along, often by the seat of my pants, but to me these medical workers were repositories of all the knowledge that I wanted.

My curiosity of veterinary medicine motivated me to spend many a day off crossing the county to Dr. Simpson's veterinary hospital where he would either take me on rounds in his truck or he would allow me to observe as he operated in his surgical facility. It was always a treat for me to learn from one of God's Directors and I would listen and ask questions. Dr. Simpson was good at letting me ask the questions and teaching without condescension even on very basic horse health subjects. We always had a good time together and some days never seemed to end. My willingness to pitch in where needed was repaid with openness to his life as a veterinarian and I liked what I saw. I was still struggling with the notion of joining the ranks of those I considered supreme beings until one day I was visiting the hospital and a surgery was planned.

Dr. Buxton was a local veterinarian in a nearby practice and he had requested the use of Dr. Simpson's surgical facility. It was the only one in the area. There was a recently castrated stallion that had developed a local infection. The scar tissue at the castration site needed to be removed surgically under anesthesia. The unwanted development is called scirrhous cord and in my decades of being a veterinarian, this is the only case I ever witnessed as it is that rare.

The two veterinarians prepared the room and the horse. There were no nurses or animal health technicians back then, only the occasional volunteer and that day, it was me. Dr. Simpson was the anesthesiologist and monitored the pulse and respiratory rates, adjusted the gas and fluids, and made sure the animal stayed asleep. Dr. Buxton draped the horse in sterile linens, set up the instruments, and scrubbed his hands before donning surgical gloves and cutting open the affected area. I was surprised at the bantering back and forth between the vets while they worked. I'm not sure what I expected, but somehow I thought it would be very serious. I became mesmerized in their surgical efficiency yet curious why, during a serious surgical procedure, the vets, especially Dr. Buxton, were telling stories and joking. The horse did not seem to care, as he lay motionless.

Suddenly, Dr. Buxton stopped and yelled to Dr. Simpson, "Do you have a catheter?"

He replied, "Yes. Why?"

Dr. Buxton said flatly, "I think I just cut the urethra."

This is the tube within the penis that carries the urine from the bladder to outside the body. Believe me, this should not be cut and would have caused numerous complications.

Dr. Simpson was already moving toward the cabinets before Dr. Buxton had answered. Locating one, he returned to the horse and under the sterile surgery drapes, placed the lubricated tube into the end of the penis and moved the tip back up toward the bladder. Dr. Buxton felt in the area of concern and upon feeling the catheter's tip pass under his fingers through the intact urethra, he sighed, "We're okay, but I think I just peed in my pants."

It was an "ah-ha moment" for me as I realized then that vets were NOT Gods and were not even close to perfect. I also realized that it was within me to become a veterinarian. These men were not that different from me after all. I knew at this point that I could do it.

Of course there are those times, the rare occurrences and instances when no matter how much knowledge you have, none of it makes a difference and that is sometimes very hard to live with.

# SHE'S GOING DOWN!

*Colic is the gastrointestinal event in horses where pain is the overt issue seen by the horse owner. The pain can range from "just not looking right" to thrashing about in the stall. Books have been written about the many causes, but in my mind I clear up the issue by categorizing them as either medical or surgical colic.*

*There are two things to remember about colic:*

*1. The degree of pain is not associated with the severity of the colic.*

*2. Time is critical between recognizing a surgical colic and getting that horse to surgery.*

*This story is about how rapid colic can come on and how, even with the best of response, it can turn out badly. My success rate with surgical colics that went to surgery was very high, about 90%. If any of my signs were met for a surgical colic - even if they were just standing there looking fine - they were shipped to surgery.*

*Today's phone call started the most dramatic colic of my career. "This is Joe at the Binghamton Dressage Facility. Are you available Doc?"*

*It was a Saturday and I was local today near my home. Telephone communication was improving and I now had a* cellular phone in my truck, but not in my pocket. I replied, "Sure Joe. What's up?"

"I'm not sure, Doc. We have a mare that isn't acting right and the trainer asked me to call you to see if you were available just in case."

My reply assured Joe that if they needed me I would be by the phone. As Joe was hanging up, I heard in the background someone yell, "She's going down!"

"Do you want me to come down Joe?"

He replied, "I guess so, but other than her going down now, she doesn't really look that bad. She ate her breakfast and the trainer just finished riding her."

I hung up the phone with the words, "I'm on my way."

The farm was an hour away but I made it in 50 minutes. The mare was being walked in the indoor arena. "Doc, if we stop walking her she just drops to the ground and rolls."

I sensed a surgical colic but wanted to do an exam before announcing this. I placed a plastic sleeve on my left arm and had them stop walking the horse so I could perform a rectal exam. My plan was to feel for an abnormality of the large intestines, which would confirm my diagnosis. However when the mare's forward progress was stopped, her legs buckled and she fell to the ground.

*We got her up and I performed the rectal as she walked. Nothing was right inside. I diagnosed torsion of the large bowel. Pulling my arm out I commanded someone to hook up a trailer. I grabbed my phone and called Cornell's answering service.*

*I cut the operator off and barked, "Sue, this is Dr. Tucker. Tell Cornell I'm bringing in a horse with surgical colic. She will be anesthetized when I arrive." Cornell and I shared the same answering service and Sue was the veteran there.*

*All she said was, "Got it," and I was gone.*

*While the mare walked, I placed a catheter in her left jugular vein and administered a large dose of sedative and some painkiller. As she slowed down, we walked her up the ramp into the large two-horse trailer with the divider and breast bars removed. This gave us enough room for her to lay down and me to remain in the stall. I quickly administered the anesthetic and she dropped onto the floor of the box stall asleep and free of pain. The back was closed. The mare and I settled in for an hour's drive to the clinic.*

*When we arrived it was clear that Sue's message had gotten to the right people. Dr. DuVries had assembled his team and they pulled the mare off the trailer onto the surgery table. Quickly cleaning and shaving her, we had her abdomen opened less than three hours from the time I had heard the words, "She's going down."*

Dr. DuVries unraveled the torsion that had rotated the colon 540 degrees – in other words the large bowel had twisted 1 and 1/2 times upon itself. The good news was that the bowel had not died so a resection or removing a piece of colon was unnecessary. The mare recovered well and settled in for a night of recovery. Her pain was gone.

During the next 24 hours interest sparked from her eyes, but early the following day, her blood became toxic in a phenomenon we didn't quite understand then.

She went into shock and died.

As veterinarians, and as horse owners, we expect that when we do everything right the results will be good. It is not always the case in a world where nature has its own set of rules.

# CHAPTER 10
*— The Tendons Were Showing —*

# CHAPTER 10

Horses are gorgeous. They are majestic. For most horse people, they are the reason for living. They complete people's lives. Thousands of books have been written to describe lives that become intertwined with an animal that has no ability to even smile. Countless words are set into rhyme and song about horses bringing every human emotion into play.

Classic movies where a horse is brought together with a leading actor have made abundant wealth for actors and producers. In the surreal world, dozens of horses have captured our sprits collectively as a population from Black Beauty to Seabiscuit.

The greatest example of connection between man and horse was evident in the year 2000 when TIME magazine ran their issue declaring the event of the Twentieth Century. They had one hundred years of items to choose from including events such as: World Wars, The Great Depression, and the emergence of technology such as mass production of cars, radios and TV, wireless phones, and even computers. We could all make a list that would take pages to identify the important moments that transformed our lives from 1901 to 2000.

TIME spent their due diligence on their list and narrowed it down to 100 moments. As I turned the pages and read each item starting at 100 and counting down, I recognized most of them. For me, the landing of men on the moon was number one; however, it was not TIME's number one.

I turned the page to reveal the number one event of the Twentieth Century and my heart stopped as gooseflesh erupted across my skin, my throat choked, and tears welled in my eyes. Secretariat! - The horse that in 1973 captured the spirit of America by winning the Triple Crown. Greatness, strength, speed, and utter domination of every racehorse that had gone before him was evident in his performances. The horse that represented the year I had started on my career had been selected as the number one moment in the world from the preceding century. To me, it spoke volumes.

During my second tour at Trotter Farm in 1976, many events occurred that shaped my destiny but they were not victories at the racetrack. Millions of people never heard about them. They were anonymous events between a horse and me. They showed me the other side of the bond between man and horse. Some of these events would thrust me beyond the normal relationship described in poetry, song, book, or movie. It was the bond of commitment, my willingness to go beyond comfort and actually be there for the horse. To give all I had without question, to cry at the end, and to move on for another.

The bond of commitment is what health care providers achieve when they are willing to help those unable to help themselves. For a veterinarian, most of the horses in need of help are there not because of their own doing, but because they are in a human's world.

Secretariat winning the Belmont Stakes by 26 lengths (you must see this on YouTube at least once before you die) is emotional and for many was a defining moment. But for me, helping the broodmare who was losing her leg while remaining a solid mother for her foal became my defining moment of commitment. I became one of those willing to help a horse no matter what the cost.

The light chestnut mare with tall hind white stockings had delivered a beautiful foal. She had become a number to the help at Mr. Trotter's barn at Trotter Farm but she carried herself with beauty and grace. This was Mr. Trotter's domain but as the assistant farm manager, I often helped with things for the two separate, but conjoined, farms.

During some point a small injury had occurred in the mare's left hind cannon area. The tiny cut had gone unnoticed by the staff. Within a few days the infection had started to spread underneath the skin and infiltrated the circulation system. The leg began to swell but the groom still didn't notice.

I suppose he no longer cared about horses or his job or family as much of his time was spent with a bottle. Ned and his family lived in a house at the farm next to Robert and his family. His tolerance for horses had long dissolved but his gentle hands remained. Ned had horseman's hands. I rarely see them today but on occasion, I'll see the soft, meaty hands with abundant kind energy glowing from the fingertips. However, Ned's hands had lost their glow from the liquor he constantly consumed. This horse suffered the consequence.

When I was asked to attend to her needs, the mare was already fighting a losing battle. The foal was not ready to be weaned and for the foal's sake, she needed to remain comfortable. This was now hard to do as the infection had spread from her hoof to above the hock. The leg had swollen to the point that the skin had burst open. The sweet smell of dead and dying tissue arose from the moist, pus covered pink layers of attempted healing. Every tendon was exposed. Fingers could be placed from one side of the limb, through the exposed tendons, and exit the other side.

"Geoff," Walt said as he pointed to the leg with a smoking cigarette wedged between his fingers, "you need to clean this up and get it wrapped."

My stomach churned at the site. The mare ate her hay as the foal lay in the deep straw. "You'll need some iodine soap and water. Clean it up good, let it dry, and wrap it to keep it clean."

"How often do I do this?" I asked.

Walt replied, "Till she dies or gets better."

For the next month I attended to her leg twice a day. Each time as I unwrapped the bandage the smell twisted my stomach. The cotton was soaked in pus and chunks of tissue clung to its fibers. I would lead the mare to a nearby hose and let her and the foal graze as I flushed the leg in cold water. She seemed to like either the pressure or the cold. I'm not sure, but whatever it was, she never complained. When the foal was hungry for milk, either side was made available without hesitation. When I was ready to clean and dress the wound, she remained motionless. I think she knew I was helping - or at least trying to. I started to connect beyond the warmth and softness of a horse's hide. I started to connect with the essence and personality of an individual horse. While this was not the first time, it was the last time of innocence for my ability and the first time I wholeheartedly committed to my calling as a veterinarian.

There is evidence that the part of the brain responsible for smells is the oldest part. Smells such as apple pie baking in the oven or a woman's perfume can trigger memories from a distant past long forgotten. For me, the sweet smell of necrotic skin brings me instantly back to that mare and the commitment I made to help horses no matter what.

As large as horses are, they can get ill quickly and die just as quickly. If a caregiver or owner is not really paying attention, or worse, just doesn't care anymore, then things can get out of hand fast. This horse with its tendons exposed was put to sleep after her foal was weaned. I will never forget this mare's courage, her willingness to rise above for her foal, and the feeling of commitment it taught me.

## Are You Drunk Yet?

*Cool, refreshing champagne flowed over my tongue and swirled down into my stomach. The poison alerted my body's defenses but there were none available to fight the onslaught. My brain was drawn to the sweet taste as the immediate buzz the alcohol created tempted my rational thoughts into submission. My empty glass extended outwards to be refilled by my jubilant mother as the clock ticked 15 minutes into the New Year.*

*While in high school at a New Year's Eve party, I drank rum and Coke into oblivion. From that point on I realized that to me, drinking alcohol was pointless. Because I did not drink, my liver had not made alcohol dehydrogenase, the enzyme required to break down alcohol into water. Any alcohol consumed by me continued to swirl in my body unchanged and fully effective in inebriating my mind. Some people call this "low tolerance" and others call this a "cheap date."*

*Twenty years later, my Mom was visiting us for the holidays. Matt was asleep and Kathy and I had invited some friends over. Mom was a party girl and to this end, had bought several bottles of the bubbly stuff. Being a vet, I knew I could be called out any time and so I firmly, and repeatedly, said, "Mom, no thanks. I don't want to drink and drive."*

*We all celebrated as midnight was reached and I could see disappointment in my mother's eyes each time she offered me champagne. At 12:15 I broke down. "Geoff," she said with a little slur to her speech and a twinkle in her eye, "no one will call now. Just one glass for me?"*

*The second glass went down easily as I enjoyed the moment. Warmth filled every part of my body as a familiar goofy grin stretch across my face. The music started to make my bones move in rhythm. I almost missed the phone making its angry noise.*

*"Geoff, this is June. My horse has colic."*

*I looked at my watch. 12:20. She lived 10 minutes away. She was also a vet and held a professor's position at Cornell. For her horse, she always used my services.*

*"I'm on my way," I said, then quickly added, "Why are you at the barn at this hour?" Was that the alcohol speaking or was I curious to find if this had been going on for hours?*

*"I just went to the barn to wish him a Happy New Year,"* she said.

*I am the poster child for not drinking and driving. That January 1st I almost became a statistic, as I was unable to keep my truck going straight down the road and between the lines. I pulled into the farm grateful I had not ditched it nor been arrested. "June!" I blurted out. "I'm a little drunk and I'm sorry."*

*June smiled and said, "I'm not worried." Her confidence in me helped to bring my swirling mind to the task of examining the horse. My head quickly cleared and sobriety soon took over. After all, it was only two glasses of champagne.*

*After diagnosing the horse with simple gas colic, I administered medication and the horse quickly returned to his normal self. I packed my gear into the truck. June gave her warmest thanks and good wishes for the New Year. As I drove away, my truck easily stayed between the lines of the road for my return home.*

*Three hundred sixty-four and a half days later, on December 31st about 9 pm, I received a call.*

*"Geoff, this is June. My boy has colic again. I thought I'd call earlier this year. Are you drunk yet?"*

# CHAPTER 11

## *— Goodbye Is Not Forever —*

# Chapter 11

The year 1977 was epic for me but when it started I had no idea the events that would unfold. It was in January, on my grandfather's deathbed that Kathy finally said yes to my marriage proposal. I had made an engagement ring by carefully winding bailing wire three times around a dowel and shaping and polishing the ends smooth. I placed it on her finger in front of him not long before he passed.

With a broad smile and tears, he said softly, "You picked a good one."

Kathy and I then went to Mom and Dad's for dinner to announce the wedding. It was a happy time that helped my dad through the loss of his father. We set the date for the end of July, 12 months after I had met Kathy in the pony barn. I didn't realize it then, but she was the missing ingredient I needed to become a veterinarian. The only facts I knew then was that Kathy had accepted my proposal of marriage, my father's father had died, and Kathy no longer worked at Trotter Farm.

It was a slow start as winter that year had been very cold and the drudgery of winter farm life tested my resolve. Kathy found a job on a nearby farm and we were able to be with each other every day. She would cook amazing meals and we would watch Star Trek on a small black and white TV. Kathy always dreamed of the future and the ability to travel where no man had gone before. I personally thought the whole show was hokie, but I loved the person next to me and so, I became a fan too. We were really living!

Spring is always very busy on a breeding farm. Working nearly around the clock meant nothing to me because I loved every minute. My education with horses grew every day and I couldn't envision anything else in my life. But this year, something was missing. I was like a young colt pawing at the stall door wanting out. I had a future with Kathy and with horses. I even had a future at Trotter Farm as their farm manager. Like the young colt, I wasn't thinking clearly. I was only in the selfish moment without clear thought of the future and what it could be. This is where Kathy's talent lay. She quietly listens to the foolishness of those around her, then with one sentence, takes someone from where they are and catapults them into the future that could be.

Her sentence to me was short and to the point. "You can do better than this."

In any person's life, no matter what good is surrounding them, the past seems to crop up to affect the present. I was a three-time college drop out. I was never successful with girls or sports or education. I had been challenged with a reading disability. Suddenly, within one year, I had found my wife and my calling to help horses. I had discovered my dyslexia and was learning how to read. I had a place to live and a solid income.

What on earth did she mean when she said I could do better than this? Were she and Dr. Simpson really right when they said I could be a veterinarian? I looked at her for a long time and said nothing. My head swirled with thoughts. One thought anchored then let go quickly being replaced with another. Slowly, like still frames of a movie starting to roll over the lens one at a time, I started to see what they saw. I realized in that moment that I would be leaving Trotter Farm, and fairly soon.

"Kathy," I said excitedly, "you're right." I held both her hands as I told her my plans. She smiled and went back to quietly listening. Her seed had been planted and she was enjoying the growth process exploding before her eyes.

I had promised Mrs. Trotter one full year and I had three more months to that commitment. Kathy, however, did not have that obligation. She and Mrs. Trotter had never gotten along. When I had made the announcement to her of my plans to marry Kathy, Mrs. Trotter was obliged to take me aside with a "facts of life" lecture about why she was the wrong person for me to marry. We sat in her orange Dodge Ram truck while the rain beat on the windows and roof. She used every trick in her book to show me that Kathy wasn't the right girl for me. She even called Kathy "mousey" which we still laugh about decades later. But it was a heavy burden that spring day when she and I had our talk. Her goal was to prevent Kathy from interfering with her plans of having me manage Trotter Farm. She filled my mind with doubt, but it was what I needed then. Contrast is always good because it brings with it clarity. With the doubt, I discovered the backbone I was developing. I started to realize that for the first time in my life I had something to fight for. I just couldn't put it into words but feelings about it came through my mind.

For my relationship with Kathy, whenever I was on the road for a few days shipping horses for the farm, all I could think of was getting back to her. I saw Kathy's face everywhere and dreamed of her homemade meatballs and spaghetti, the first meal she had ever made me. I even realized that my dog E-Z was as comfortable with her when I was away as he was with me. This was a sure sign that I needed to fight for her and our future together.

My meeting with Mrs. Trotter ended without her victory but its importance was not yet measured in my win column. That would come much later.

I came to the realization that I could no longer stay at the farm. I became open to leaving even though I wasn't sure where I would go. Willie, who owned the local horse transportation business, became my exit strategy. Willie was as tall as me but half my waist size. His one lazy eye made it difficult to look at him while talking. There was always a lit cigar somewhere and a beer close by. His body was stiff from wear but his movement across the ground was as smooth as a swan crossing a lake. He made friends with everyone but if you didn't like him, he just didn't care. A long puff on the well-chewed cigar and a brief, "Screw 'em then!" with a big grin, and off he would go to do something else.

Willie liked me and knew I was a good driver though he had never seen me drive. He just assumed that if Mrs. Trotter kept using me as her van driver, I must be good. One afternoon, he approached me on the farm and said, "Hey Geoff! You want to start driving for me? If you say yes, I'll have you in Nevada next week."

My opening was set. I had a job that paid real money with a future wife whose job included an apartment. I would be set, but that darned integrity thing got in the way. I had promised a full year and the foaling season wasn't over. I had to ask Willie if that offer could wait until June.

Willie quickly answered, "You bet."

With that, I started to float. Driving 18-wheelers for a living was a life that just could not get any better.

I gave Mrs. Trotter my notice for June 1st, exactly 12 months from my hire date and almost 3 months away. Kathy and I continued to make wedding plans for July and in my spare time I went on calls with Dr. Simpson. I was still hooked on horses and I asked him during my travels to farms what I should do next as far as perusing a veterinary career.

Dr. Simpson's advice was simple, "Go to Cornell."

"But it will cost too much. I don't have the money," I said.

He replied, "Geoff, don't worry about the money. There are ways to get the money."

"But I don't have the grades," I said defending my position with another excuse.

He replied, "It's not just grades. It's your experience plus who you know." He continued to teach me additional facts of life that my parents and Mrs. Trotter had not mentioned. "Look," he said as he pulled the truck up to a farm, "these guys that determine if you get into Cornell are just humans. They play golf. They ask each other if you know so and so. If they know you, they'll say "Sure I know Geoff Tucker! You should let him in." That's the way it goes. It's not just the grades."

He then gave me a few names of local veterinarians he thought I should meet and promised to write me a letter of recommendation for admission. We got out of the truck but I can't remember much else of that day. At night with Kathy I told her what was said. She nodded with understanding and then said, "You should talk to those other veterinarians."

The inside of a man's brain, at least this man's brain, is a very confusing place and strangers should never enter it without knowing the risk they take of being chopped up and spat out. Kathy was either oblivious to this risk or she was totally unafraid. The scissors of thoughts cut through my brain matter as I started to realize that I was about to walk down the path where I was totally lying to everyone I would meet. Out of my mouth would sound words such as, "Yes, I am planning to attend veterinary school and will become an equine veterinarian in the future." However, my mind was saying, "You can't read, you hate tests, you've failed school several times. What are you doing?" To this day I cannot tell you how I overcame my doubts and fears. Kathy's confidence played a huge part, but I also think it was a feeling of "why not" as I confronted the absurdity of the whole process. Like a soldier marching into a battle of insurmountable odds, I called and met with several local vets and started my application process to Cornell undergraduate school.

By July, I was driving tractor-trailer trucks back and forth to Kentucky or Virginia and once to Florida. I became very good at this. I quickly became a solo driver earning more money and living very well. I have many great memories made in this short time. I continued to use my eyes as a shutter memorizing license plates and graduating up to exit signs and billboards. I started to read more confidently. I also had my eyes examined and glasses prescribed for my vision. Another unusual finding was made that showed that my left eye was better at reading things close up but my right eye was better for distance. My night vision was and still is excellent. I can read anything upside down like the newspaper in front of the person facing me at the breakfast table. The eyes are a direct extension of the brain and there was nothing normal about my brain. I should have expected the eyes to follow suit.

July 23rd came fast and I went to Amsterdam, New York. I had a shot of whiskey and chugged a beer chaser with my best friend from high school and now best man. Twenty minutes later I stood at the altar as I watched my bride walk down the aisle towards me. The party went most of the night but we escaped before sunset and headed east. Glouster, Massachusetts became our honeymoon destination and we became tourists thoroughly enjoying our new lives as Mr. and Mrs. Tucker. We had no cares in the world.

A short time later, I found myself back behind the wheel of my truck heading to a barn in Watertown, Connecticut. This was still a world without cell phones and I was surprised at the farm to get a message from my dispatcher telling me to turn around and head back home. My father had just been taken to the hospital.

Calmness prevailed as I drove the hour back to the shop. Another 45 minutes passed as I traveled to the apartment Kathy and I shared. It took another hour as I helped her finish up preparing the horses for her early departure. Finally we got cleaned up and found the hospital my father had been taken to. He was on the commuter train from New York City when he had his heart attack, stopping the train in a strange city.

In January, when my grandfather was on his deathbed, I saw my dad swallow some pills. "What are those for, Dad?" I asked.

"Oh, these? They are nitroglycerin. My doctor has me taking these for my heart."

"Why?" I was concerned.

My dad deflected my concerned tone by simply saying, "Oh, he's a little worried about something he saw on a test he gave me. It's really nothing to worry about."

Now, six months later, I saw him lying in a bed, unconscious, with tubes sprouting from his arms and face. I would never get to talk with him again. He died during the night three weeks after my wedding, and one day before

Elvis Presley died. It seemed absolutely surreal and the loss took days to make it to my consciousness. I felt alone.

I lay awake in my bed three days after he was gone. My wife sleeps lightly and wakes for the slightest thing but I sleep soundly through everything. Kathy's Airedale dog, Casey, never made a noise and my E-Z would bark at everything. That night I woke to Casey's moaning as he lay at the bottom of the stairs. My eyes shot open. "Kathy, do you hear that?" I asked, but she remained sound asleep. E-Z was motionless with eyes closed and his paws twitched to his doggie dream of chasing some invisible intruder. I rose to the sitting position.

I didn't breathe and just listened. Casey moaned again then became silent. There in our bedroom a presence appeared as clear to me as the keyboard under my fingertips as I write this. It was my father. He simply said, "We didn't have a chance to say good-bye. I wanted to let you know, I'm all right." He smiled and waited for me to smile. As tears formed he said goodbye and rose out of my presence. There was no more howling from Casey.

Kathy and E-Z awoke. She asked, "What's wrong?"

I told her that Dad had just come to say good-bye. Kathy knew that it was true as I lay back down and fell deeply asleep.

I now knew the support I was receiving from those around me and those I met and so I moved forward with my application to Cornell. The forms were filled out and the package sent. I waited and was very quickly rewarded with a letter saying they were interested in accepting me BUT.... Memories of the past rose to the surface as visions of rejection letters showed their ugly words.

With a jolt, Kathy said, "But... what?"

"Cornell wants me to take some courses to see if I can handle their curriculum. They suggest a science and a math course." I felt dejected, but my Dad's recent visit bolstered my spirits. Then with conviction I said, "Great! I'll go to the local community college and enroll in their night classes."

A few days later I was at Pace College in Valhalla, NY enrolling in a basic science course and calculus. Willie helped me by scheduling my driving times around my night classes. I studied everywhere and all the time. I took the tests and passed. I felt my dad and grandfather both help me during the process. My final grades in November were A's.

I sent my transcripts off to Cornell and again waited. On the day before Christmas I opened the thin official letter from the University. A thin letter in my experience meant rejection. My wife sat close and held my arm. I read, and then read again. Tears formed and I choked as I tried to read the words to her.

Kathy grabbed the paper from me and read it herself. Throwing her arms up in the air and then around me, she cried out, "I knew you could do it!" followed quickly with her shouting, "We're moving to Ithaca!"

# LONG HOT DOG DAYS OF SUMMER

*The summer heat could blister paint. Dogs that normally chased my truck onto the farm lay motionless in the shade moving only their eyes assessing the trespasser, and then drifting off to a sleep where it was cooler and they were chasing rabbits again. Whines and gently puffing cheeks along with flicking paws were evidence of their deep sleep. "If only I were a dog," I thought as I went into the barn for another routine call.*

*August days in upstate New York can be brutally hot. Life creeps by in inches. I worked my way through the morning calls. A pregnancy check, an insurance exam, and a few Coggins tests and health certificates, all not too stressful for me so far. It was almost noon and I had a lameness exam next.*

*Standing outside in the sun for an hour, I watched the slightly lame horse move around in a circle. He was lame mostly to the right and I did the usual exams of hoof testers, flexion tests, and nerve blocks. The results yielded gallons of sweat pouring off my eyebrows and chin. My shirt was soaked.*

189

I went to the truck to get the heavy X-ray machine and bulky film plates and set everything up. Another 30 minutes of pulling the shoes, preparing the hoof and packing the sole with Play-Doh™ to help clarify the bone structures within the hoof, I neared exhaustion. The horse was just beyond cooperation, as he would move the hoof out of position just before I would trigger the X-ray for the exposure. Frustration was hard to keep in check.

The exam was over and my equipment was packed again in the truck. My sweat-drenched clothes added 20 pounds to my weight and stuck to the hot seats. I quickly drove to the local "Red Apple" convenience store and nosed my truck up tightly to a big tree. The shade covered the cab of my truck. I turned up the music, made the air conditioning cold, cracked the window open, and tilted the back of the seat as far as it would go. Moments later I joined the same world the dogs I had seen earlier in a deep, deep sleep.

I felt nothing and my brain waves were flat lined. I could have been dead. I left my body and I could not even tell you what I was experiencing. I was in a pure state of nothingness. My body maintained this state long enough to be rejuvenated, but something was wrong. It told me to wake up immediately, but forgot to tell me who I was or where I was.

My eyes opened but my body had no feeling of the surroundings and my mind was blank. My arms lay limp at my sides and my legs had fallen widely apart. My lips could not *move. Slowly my eyes focused. I saw the tree directly in front of me. I was about to die.*

*Screaming at the top of my lungs, I lifted both of my legs and slammed them on the brakes crushing the peddle into the floorboard. I braced for impact, but nothing happened. My conscious brain started to analyze things. My screaming had stopped. Music gently wafted in the cool air. I looked around hoping no one had heard my screaming.*

*After a few moments had passed, I slipped the gear from park to reverse and backed away from the shade tree and out of the parking lot. Heading to my afternoon appointment, I started laughing out loud. In a parked truck, I had thought my life was going to have a horrible end. It is a feeling I have never forgotten and gives me the giggles every time the long hot dog days of summer meets the late afternoon drooping eye lids.*

# CHAPTER 12

*— A New Beginning —*

# CHAPTER 12

New Year's Day in 1978 was cold and the skies drained every snowflake they could produce upon Westchester County, New York. No one traveling on the holiday created quietness in the countryside. The blanket of snow dampened any sound to silence. Nursing hangovers or making family breakfasts or pondering resolutions was the order of the day for most citizens. Kathy and I, however, had other plans. The van was packed with every earthly belonging we owned. So was the Kruger car.

The Krugers' family had been friends with my family forever. Ted, the father, was a Cornell alumnus and when he had heard I had been accepted, he took over the father role in my life and declared his help in moving us to Ithaca. We had chosen this day without thinking of the unpredictable weather of January in New York.

The trip took twice as long as we had expected but we arrived safely. Kathy and I had visited Ithaca just after Christmas to find an apartment, which today was waiting for our vanload of furniture and belongings. We went to dinner that night and celebrated my start toward becoming a veterinarian. I was excited, but my mind swirled with past educational failures – and there were so many! This was not a trade school or even a meager liberal arts school. This was an Ivy League University. Here was my wife, my mom, and my surrogate dad and mom all sitting around me and I was torn between elation and fear. I suppose everyone has the jitters like this but I know mine were worse. Not only did I not want to let them down, I didn't' want to let myself down. This was my dream and I couldn't fail – not this time.

Cornell University is made of several colleges put together each with their own campuses. Where I went to school is hardly recognizable today, as the university has built structures everywhere. Back in 1978, it was still larger than any school I had ever attended. It was intimidating. Immediately I missed the openness and quiet of the farm and being with horses every moment. Now I lived in a row of one-bedroom apartments, one of 5 buildings in the middle of a beef farm. Thoughts of meeting my advisor, selecting courses, and finding my way around campus filled my time.

My purpose of going back to college was to learn everything I could about horses. I believed that the answer to the question of why horses curl up their noses when you scratch their withers was in a book somewhere. I was now at an institution of higher learning where all the answers would become available to me, or so I thought. With this in mind I combed all the schedules for classes about horses. Finding only three classes, I reviewed the booklets again. There was one listed class about horse genetics, for upperclassmen and by appointment only, and was given by my advisor. Another was a course that was not just about horses. The third was Horse 265 offered to 2nd and 3rd year students. That was it.

I went to my advisor where he confirmed this lack of horse classes. He then advised me that to get into veterinary school, horse classes were not important. Prerequisites included microbiology, organic chemistry, physiology, biochemistry, as well as speech and debate and several animal science courses including animal reproduction and animal nutrition. I became excited with the thoughts of learning all this new information, and then quickly became overwrought with the fear of my experience with marine microbiology. I saw myself writing, "Out to lunch" again on my tests. I agreed on my first set of classes and went home very uncertain about how things would go.

I went over my day with Kathy but only showed my excitement and not my fears. It was easy to do because I had purchased many new books and the excitement of my young days came back with the new book smells.

Kathy mentioned that we needed money and she was starting to look for a job. The logistics of being newlyweds living in an off campus apartment with one vehicle and two independent schedules started to creep into my consciousness. The exact mechanisms we employed aren't clear; we just did what we had to do and that feeling of determination to make it happen remains today. Things started off fine, then the February snowstorm came. Walking the two dogs was my job and the snow that day was above my waist. A good snowfall is fun, but at some point over time it merely exists to make humans and animals miserable and so it was that winter. Never in the next 18 years in Ithaca did it ever snow as much as it did that month. It was almost as if someone was testing our resolve, but we persevered.

Money was always an issue and I spent much of my academic days filling out government forms for financial aid. Part of that aid included work-study programs where employment was made available for students. Working at Cornell's Equine Research Park was the coveted position for those wanting to work with horses and of course, as a new student, was virtually impossible for me to get. Many jobs included caring for lab rats but I had my standards. I had cleaned stalls for two full years already and had advanced to assistant farm manager of a Thoroughbred breeding and training farm. I had driven a million dollars of horseflesh all over the United States in 18-wheelers. I was not going to clean rat cages.

Soon an opening occurred at the Equine Isolation Facilities. These two long barns were situated far above the campus and my job was to care for the isolated ponies on the weekend. The two men I worked for were Dr. Keener and Dr. Conyers. They both were world renowned for their research with horses and their work was regarded as gospel. In fact, every horseman knows of Dr. Conyer's work, but they would not know it outright. This was perfect for me because I could start to network with these esteemed veterinary researchers so when they played golf they could tell the others about me. My first day was exciting.

I arrived at the barn Saturday morning at 7 am and was met by another full time worker who said, "Let me show you the ropes." We went into the first building that involved opening one set of doors, walking through an empty foyer, and then walking through another set of doors. This led into a brightly fluorescent-lit hallway lined with beige colored painted glazed cinder blocks and ceiling. It reminded me of a prison. Brown metal doors were the only appointments to the hallway and dark tile covered the floor. Clean but not sterile described this part of the building. The worker and I together entered the first door on the left. He closed the door behind us.

We were in a very small room no bigger than a large closet. Hanging on the wall were two sets of green coveralls and on the floor were two pairs of black rubber boots. We put them on, stepped into the disinfectant footbath, then opened the other door from that room and walked into the animal area. The door was closed behind us. We were now in the pathogen free section.

The animal area had two parts. The first was the 10 x 10 foot stall where the pony stood and the second was the 5 x 5 foot work area where the equipment was kept. He said, "Your job is simple. Take the pony's rectal temperature and record it on the chart. Feed the pony the food that has been prepared there in the bags. Take the hose and wash down the floor so all the manure and urine are gone. Clean up the equipment area, go back into the prep room and wash the boots, take the boots and coveralls off, leave this one station and go to the next. Repeat this for every station in the building. Got it?"

The smell, while not offensive, was indescribable in terms a horseman would understand. The atmosphere was sterile. The air in the building was drawn out and fresh air was sent through an expensive filter so the smell was best described as nothing. There was no bedding of any kind. Hay was pre-measured and every strand was usually gone. Buckets were cleaned every day and the floor washed with high-pressure water. The floor was sealed in hard rubber. This was what these ponies lived in for the term of the experiment.

Most of the ponies used in these conditions were tractable by the poorest of horsemen, but a few were difficult. Taking rectal temperatures was difficult. Catching them often proved to be the task of the day. On one lonely Sunday morning as I went to remove the thermometer, the

199

pony clamped his tail as I pulled on the string that attached the glass tube to the tail clip. The string came off and the thermometer was sucked into the pony. I was on the job for about a month and had never seen another soul of authority. It was always me along with another student. We would do the morning chores then sit at a table in the lunchroom of the main building and study or sleep. In the afternoon we would repeat the morning chores then go home at four. The ponies would be left until 7 am the next morning.

I went to the emergency call list and called the person on duty. I was told to go back often to check the pony. He said the thermometer would fall out in the next pile of manure and not to worry. It did breaking into a thousand pieces with mercury pooling into those droplets we used to play with when we were kids. Today a haz-mat team would have been called. On that Sunday, it was just a blip in the day.

I often would lay awake at night thinking of the lives these ponies were living. Solitude away from all other horses living on hard rubber floors and no exposure to the world a horse knows and loves. When the experiment was over they were returned to the pony herd and allowed to be ponies. Some however were used constantly because they were well behaved and easy to work with. Some died in captivity during an experiment. Though it was hard, I slowly learned to block it out when the day was done. Over the years as a vet working with horses I would be exposed to things like this that treated the horse as anything but a horse. From outright starvation to horses just leading quiet lives of desperation to horses that were made surrogate humans for their owners, I have seen it all. It was here at the isolation units I learned to dissociate from these abominations. I had to in order to learn to work with all horses where they were and not be caught up in emotion. If I let my emotions take over, I couldn't help the other horses. Focusing on the bad only limited my ability to attend to those who really needed care with owners willing to get it.

The work at the isolation units also exposed me to the fallacy that science experimentation is exact and good. This happened on a Saturday morning when I took the first pony's temperature and it was over 103. I don't know why, but I left the stall and went to the other ponies and saw they were also lethargic. I took several more temperatures and they were all significantly elevated. I called the boss, Dr. Conyers. His immediate concern was evident as he asked me questions. He then said he would be out immediately. In a short time he and Dr. Keener arrived and we went through each pony with the same results. Apparently this was a reaction to an experiment done earlier in the week. Somehow, the few ponies in the experiment were not the only ones affected. Somehow there was a break in the system and every pony was affected. Much head scratching went on that day.

Lessons learned from observation of life going on around you sometimes are more valuable than words written in a text. My brief time in the Equine Isolation Units taught me lessons carried forward throughout my career. Scientific experimentation is not always accurate or reliable. What we do in the name of scientific experimentation is not glorious to the animals or their keepers. I left this job as soon as I could. Dr. Keener and I became acquaintances at future veterinary get-togethers and he became an advocate for my admission to the vet school. I was still heading in the right direction, though my path's rose-colored glasses were becoming tainted with reality.

I couldn't wait for summer vacation. We were broke and I wasn't learning anything I thought was important for my future. I passed all my classes but it was a struggle. It was time to stop and refresh for a while. Ithaca was beautiful, but I negotiated a two-week stint with my old horse-hauling outfit to drive, which I did as much as I could without taking away from the full time drivers.

I had met Dr. Jackson before traveling south for the summer and tried to get a job at The Equine Research Park where he was the director. It hadn't happened that summer but I was on the list for the fall. I did what I could to make money and so did Kathy. She got a job at Olin Mills Photography Studio as one of those annoyances that called you at you dinner hour asking you to buy their services. She hated it. By the time the fall came around, she decided to also matriculate and Cornell said, "Sure, why not?" After all she had completed her associate's degree at Delhi University and had always done well in school.

Kathy would attend some of the same animal science class as I did. She would sit there listening to the lecture while I wrote down everything the professor said. Taking no notes, she would take the test and get a B or better after studying one night while I would study for days, get sick, and muddle out with a B- or worse. She made it look so easy.

I also needed to work on another plan because my grades weren't going to get me into vet school. I struggled with all my classes and became frustrated that there were so few courses on horses. I decided to do something about it. I started a horse club and called it The Cornell Student's Horsemen's Association. I needed permission from the head of the Animal Science Department and I also needed a professor to advise the group. I was told to ask Dr. Heinrich who eventually became a friend and strong supporter of my future endeavors. He agreed and posters went up announcing the first meeting.

We met on a Thursday night and there were about 30 students along with Dr. Heinrich sitting looking at me. The adrenaline raced through my sweat glands and forced my voice into a quivering falsetto. This was my first public speaking event and I never realized I would be in this position, in front of a group of people, until I was in front of them. I stared at the audience as fear gripped me. Kathy smiled back with a confident energy and I opened my mouth and started speaking.

I laid out the structure of the meeting and our purpose and elected myself as president and asked for others to become other officers. I then announced that there were a few rules to follow. One rule however was unusual and Dr. Heinrich smiled as I said it. I announced that it was "legal" that no matter who was speaking, at any time, anyone could stand up and announce a "five-minute spiel." This applied even if a guest speaker was talking. It was bold and the idea caught on. I then did the first five-minute spiel as I discussed some research a biomechanics engineer was doing with force plate technology and horse gaits. It was a lot of research to cram into five minutes, but it was fun. The association got off to a good start.

During the next year I pursued the expansion of The Cornell Student Horsemen's Association. The New York State 4-H was headquartered in the Animal Science building and Dr. Samuels ran this. The truth really was that Judy, his secretary, did all the work and she became such a valuable friend as she often doubled as my secretary. I don't think I ever thanked her enough.

One of the things the 4-H did was to host the state finals of Horse Bowl. This was a competition between two teams of four members each. The teams would sit on either side of a moderator who would ask a horse related question such as, "How many legs does a horse have?" Players had an electronic button in front of them and the first to press the button would cause the moderator to stop reading. The person with the light on in front of them would answer the question. If answered correctly, the team would get a point. The first to reach 20 points would win the round.

I became involved with this because of a vet student who also lived in the apartments in the cow field where we lived. Her name was Jesse and we would spend countless nights writing the questions used in these competitions. With stacks of books to use for verification, we would learn all there was known about horses. This was before Trivial Pursuit or the Internet where information was right at your fingertips. This not only was a fun way to learn for me, but it was very serious competition for the kids throughout the state.

I thought it would be a great idea to expand this to the college level. I started to contact the department chairs of all the Agricultural schools in New York to propose the creation of the Intercollegiate Horse Bowl competition. There was reluctance from several schools, but I wasn't sure why. I finally persuaded three schools and then pitting their acceptance against the resistant schools, which virtually forced them to also join the party.

Our team at Cornell was serious and we had many nights writing questions and studying. We assumed the other schools did too. However, it was a rout as we easily won the first competition. We visited the other schools and some worked hard to get better as they were competitive. I was surprised though that several other schools folded quickly feeling they weren't as smart as Cornell students. I was naive thinking we were all as interested in learning as much as we could about horses. I became aware that my fellow students were fierce competitors all fighting for admission to veterinary school while the agriculture students weren't as driven. It was the beginning of my realization that not all students are created equal. I was also realizing that maybe I wasn't so stupid after all even though I was still struggling with my classes.

Over the winter, I concentrated even more on my studying. We were poor, and it was cold again but we were where we wanted to be, doing what we wanted to do. Kathy and I were both hired by The Equine Research Park in the spring and were excited on our first day at work. Like with the isolation units, students were hired to do weekend chores. The park was laid out with several barns each with a number of animals that needed to be turned out for exercise, fed, and to have stalls cleaned. An experienced student met us and taught us the routine.

Kathy and I were shocked with what we were told. The first rule was that no horse was to be handled. Chutes made of gates or unrolled wire fencing framed with wood boards were stretched between the barn and the paddock gates. Once in place, the horses were turned loose and allowed to run, often slipping on cement or bumping into objects as the wild pack screamed for the outdoors. Foals and yearlings were not haltered and led. Two year olds had not been trained to lead.

We then were told to pick out the stalls into the gutter cleaner where the manure was moved from the converted dairy barn into a spreader where it was left for the Monday employee to dump. Some shavings were lightly covered over the wet spots. Work that started at 7 am and was done by 10 am in such a poor fashion that both Kathy and I said to each other, "Not on our watch!"

Against the direct orders of Dr. Jackson, we started to teach the horses how to lead during our first weekend of work. In addition we thoroughly cleaned every stall. Our day started around 6:30 am and would not stop until about 4 pm. Our work we thought went unnoticed, but there were eyes everywhere. Harold and Alice lived on the farm and silently witnessed everything. Harold was the retired farrier at Cornell and taught many farriers at the vet's farrier school. He also taught me all that I know about the horse's foot later on, but at this point, he and his wife were just observing.

One weekend Dr. Jackson came out and caught us leading the young horses and became upset with us. With the thoughts of going to vet school hanging on what I said, I looked at him and apologized but then added that Kathy and I did this for a living for years and NOT leading them was dangerous. With that, Kathy and I continued to lead the rest of the horses in a safe and controlled manor. He saw the wisdom in what we were doing and a friendship started between us lasting to this day.

The foaling season had started and many of the vet school's horses were at the Research Park. Dr. Mann and Dr. Donovan were in charge of this part of the operation. Kathy and I were working a lot and had become very close with the horses. Both Dr. Mann and Dr. Donovan had determined that one of the mares due to deliver soon was not going to foal that night according to their exams. From my foaling experience at Trotter Farm I was sure that she was about to deliver. It was subtle and hard to explain, but I said to Kathy that she was going tonight.

We decided to stay up all night at the park just to watch. This is something Kathy and I had done a lot the last spring before going back to college. We would both camp out in the barn. I would usually sleep soundly but Kathy would hear the horse's water break and wake me. We together witnessed the miracle of birth on numerous occasions. Tonight at the Equine Research Park we were going to do it again.

I talked two other students into joining us. Kathy was the first to leave. She said she believed me but she was going to sleep in a bed that night and I was on my own. She left about 10 pm. Maria was the next to leave about 1 am and Jim left at 3 am. Both of these students were also pre-veterinary and while Maria got in, Jim did not. He was a good guy and would have made a good vet, but his wife was not as supportive as Kathy and I really believe that support at home creates a synergy that is vitally important.

It was 5 am when the mare finally laid down and pushed out the foal. There was a problem in that the stall door had a gap of about a foot between the door bottom and the floor. The mare had positioned her back end against this gap and the foal was delivered onto the barn aisle outside of the stall. With little effort, I opened the door and dragged the newborn into the stall. Assured that all was well with mom and baby, I bicycled over to the vet school cafeteria. I was angry.

I found Dr. Jackson sitting at a table drinking coffee with other vet students. I walked up to him with a piece of mind I needed to vent. I declared that the mare foaled.

His reply was, "I hate people who say I told you so."

Being without sleep and hungry and after witnessing again the ineptitude of what I had thought to be the top in education in horses, I let loose.

"Dr. Jackson," I said mustering up courage to speak to someone I thought I should show respect to. "I stayed up to be sure all went well with this foaling. It is important to attend these events because bad things can happen and it did last night. She delivered the foal under the door and into the aisle. The help would not have arrived until 7 am and that foal could have died and the frantic mare could have become injured." I stopped for a moment to catch my breath. Realizing that I probably in a moment had lost any opportunity to get into vet school, I continued with a what-the-heck attitude.

Dr. Jackson was speechless, as he knew I wasn't done. "Furthermore," I proclaimed with a finger pointing somewhere to make a point, "I am starting a foal watch group with the students of the Horsemen's Association. We will take turns watching every delivery this spring and will call you or Dr. Mann when a mare starts to deliver." With a quick, "Thank you" from my lips I ended this authoritative one-sided confrontation with the man who I thought was my only ticket into my dreams. I turned and walked away not waiting for a reply. My heart started beating once again with resounding thuds in my ears.

Before the next foal hit the ground, Foal Watch became a focus of the CSHA and several lucky students saw their first foaling. We even included vet students who wanted to join. I still struggled with biochemistry and physiology but I was starting to have fun. By the time summer break came, Kathy and I had full time jobs at the research park with seniority. The grumpy old Harold had warmed up and he started to show me things about horse's feet that would last until today. Dr. Jackson assigned me to special projects worthy of an undergraduate. Overall, I was starting to feel accepted by the people I thought were important in the progression of my career. More importantly, I was starting to add to the Cornell community and they were listening.

## BLACK WALNUTS ON A BLACK NIGHT

*My body had been relaxing after dinner and I was feeling warm and content when the phone rang. It was a Friday evening in November a week after Thanksgiving. The caller said that both of her horses weren't feeling well. I told her I would be there in 30 minutes, layered myself in warm clothes, and headed out to my truck.*

*The temperatures were hovering at the freezing mark and while the night was crystal clear, the new moon shed no light on the roads I was driving on. Arriving at the barn on schedule, I found the door in the dark and entered into the warm glow of the pair of low wattage incandescent bulbs in the ceiling. The glow was warm but the temperature was still bone chilling.*

The two Trottingbred ponies quietly stood in cross ties, one behind the other. I started my routine of temperature, pulse, and respiration. I asked questions. Nothing made sense. The ponies were depressed, but that was it for signs of a disease. It was time for the rectal exam which I took my time doing. This helped warm my arm as well as gave me time to think. The first pony gave me nothing to work with, but the second one did.

My left arm was fully inserted in the rectum of the second pony and my right hand gently rested on its back. As I struggled to put the pieces together, I started to look around the barn. My eyes, straining in the darkness, saw two clear plastic bags about three feet in diameter and four and a half feet tall. "What are those," I asked?

"Those bags are my stall shavings," she said.

"Where did you get them?" I asked as I withdrew my arm.

Proudly she replied, "I got them yesterday from the local furniture mill. They were free!"

I opened one bag and saw the hardwood shavings that look so different from the normal light tan to yellow pine shavings. I sniffed to confirm the lack of pine smell. These had the different smell of a furniture factory and a dark color.

My solution had appeared from the shadows. I drew up some medications and started to explain. "Those shavings have *black walnut in them which usually cause little problems in ponies, but in horses they can cause severe founder. Your horses are between ponies and horses so they must be more susceptible to the effects than Shetland ponies."*

*In 1983, several horses mysteriously became lame at a farm in Bedford Hills, NY. Many of those horses died from severe and acute laminitis - also known as founder. This is when the bone inside the hoof detaches from the hoof wall causing excruciating pain. These horses were autopsied at the Cornell Veterinary School and a team of vets from that school went to investigate the farm.*

*The investigation revealed that the farm had bought bulk shavings from a furniture maker. Black walnut trees were used in the laminating process and in finishing the furniture, shavings of that tree were created. The team of veterinarians and students performed tests on ponies and horses. Shavings as well as extracted juglone were used to replicate the disease. Juglone is the chemical the black walnut tree excretes to kill all vegetation growing around it that improves the chances of young black walnut plants to grow without competition.*

*The results of all the research done back then was that for some unknown reason, horses and not ponies who are stalled on shavings made with black walnut trees in a laminating furniture plant will severely founder. This still remains a mystery today.*

*It was black walnuts on a black night that almost killed these ponies. If the bags had been kept in another room or if I hadn't paused while doing my rectal exam to look about the room, these ponies could have severely foundered. Instead, luck was with them and they fully recovered.*

# CHAPTER 13

*— Frustrated and Broke —*

# CHAPTER 13

That Spring I had started the Cornell Student Horseman's Association, the Intercollegiate Horse Bowl competition, and Foal Watch. In addition, I had passed all the classes including Horses 265. I'll admit I did not get an A in the only class devoted to horses. I didn't even get a C in Organic chemistry, although I did get an A in Organic Chemistry Lab where I made wintergreen and other interesting things.

I was frustrated. I was working as hard as I could in my classes and I had little to show for it. We were working our butts off at the Equine Research Park. We were low on cash. We applied for government food stamps – a new low. We were miserable but committed to finishing the process. I had to wonder if this would be worth it. I had seen so much before going to Cornell and now it appeared that I was just wasting my time doing busy work and not learning much in my classes that applied to horses. In addition, students that had done nothing with their lives other than to go to school and bury their heads in books surrounded me. They knew little about horses and couldn't really hold an intelligent conversation about a given horse topic so we didn't have much to chat about.

I was at a university where I thought they would have all the answers and all they had were more books and next to nothing about horses in those books. Their horse programs and facilities were staffed with people that seemed only to care about them Monday through Friday from 7 am to 4 pm like they were objects or things, not living animals. The professors were not horsemen bringing years of experience to the teaching venue, but rather they were gifted scientists that looked at horses more as a training opportunity and not in terms of having any sort of connection to a human.

At the Research Park the vet students were some of the worst weekend help there was. If they had worked on any horse farm I'd ever been at they'd have been fired the first week. They only did the minimum and then disappeared from the farm. The horses lived in their own waste for two days and were never seen from 3 pm when they left till 8 am the next day when they showed up late. Kathy and I felt helpless and the situation encouraged us to do more on the weekends we were assigned to work. We became shocked when their irresponsible behavior was never punished but rather condoned.

In this state of frustration I buried my head in my pillow and drifted off to sleep. The morning sun emerged into my consciousness waking me from a place where ideas stir and form at night. I sat upright in bed electrified with resolve. "Kathy!" I said without regard to her sleep state.

"What?" came from somewhere inside a pillow.

"I have this great idea! I am going to send all these students to Kentucky to see real horse farms!" I was excited and was expecting Kathy's enthusiastic reply.

Instead she said, "How you gonna do that?"

"I'm going to have a weekend symposium and with the proceeds, I will send them. I'll call it the "I Love New York Horse Symposium" and I'll use the heart symbol just like the state does."

With that, I went to work with a renewed vigor and Kathy jumped in full force with me. I presented this idea to the Association and to Dr. Heinrich. I asked for volunteers to help get things started. I specifically asked for some summer volunteers. I also asked Judy from Dr. Samuel's office for help.

I put together people I thought would be great speakers. They were divided into two groups: faculty and non-faculty. The faculty was easy. I found a weekend in November 1979 when there were no conflicts then I personally asked for their commitment. I told them they would be paid nothing and this seemed to be understood as no problem.

Then we focused on the non-faculty. I asked the head of Fasig-Tipton, the largest Thoroughbred sales company in the world, and he agreed. I asked an attorney from California who had just written a book of *Law for the Horse Owner*. He agreed to fly from California at his own expense to come speak. I asked the father of blood typing and horse identification to speak and he said yes. I asked a revered professor in Ohio to speak on lameness and he said yes. The subjects covered not only medicine, but they also covered taxes for horsemen, riding for the handicapped, poisonous plants, and careers in the horse industry. Kathy and I started advertisements for the program and the first check arrived at Judy's office soon after.

We were all excited at this point. "We" being Kathy, Judy, and I. Every other volunteer had failed on their assignments as they headed off to summer commitments so Kathy and I became absorbed in putting together the program single handedly and in doing so, we forgot to keep our advisor abreast of the details. Dr. Heinrich believed in laissez-faire up to a point but we were burning through our allocated school funds with little accountability.

Kathy and I were walking west from the vet school toward the Animal Science building on the north side of the road and Dr. Heinrich was heading in the opposite direction on the south side. He saw us and with a look of worry on his face, motioned for us to cross the street and join him for an impromptu street meeting. His large forehead wrinkled as he said in a most serious tone, "Geoff, it's getting toward the end of summer and I'm worried that things may not be progressing on the symposium project." Kathy and I glanced at each other, instantly realizing our mistake, and burst out laughing - literally. We both had been out of school and saddled with so many responsibilities that we had forgotten that Dr. Heinrich worked with high school kids who may be brilliant, but who also did not know the responsibility of commitment. As a bewildered smile crept across his face, Dr. Heinrich moved to a position between worry and relief, but he wasn't sure. His eyes asked for an explanation and I eagerly filled him in on all the plans that had come together. I listed the committed speakers, the commitment of the vet school auditorium and the clearance of the use of their campus for part of the event. I started to throw out the items on our to-do list scheduled for completion between today and the beginning of school. By the time I was done, Dr. Heinrich was doing the jig all the way back to his office. He forgot why he was out on the street in the first place.

The first meeting of the CSHA in September was filled with excitement as the members started to volunteer: shopping for refreshments, becoming taxi drivers for speakers, badges, and so on. The checks kept pouring in from as far away as Massachusetts and Ohio. With the event only days away, we were all in high gear. We had split the venue between the vet school and the animal science building. We had reserved campus busses to shuttle people from the parking lot. We had thought of everything. At least we felt confident.

Saturday morning came with beautiful autumn upstate NY weather. I had not slept a wink. People started to arrive and we had students everywhere to act as guides. More people came. Excitement rose. Faculty members arrived and felt the excitement and energy as they mingled with the crowd. The guest speakers came in with a presence demanding their importance. It was not until 10 minutes before the start that my nerves became frayed. I was to get up in front of over 500 paying attendees plus faculty, students, and guest speakers and open my mouth.

As my heart pounded in an attempt to save my life from the attacking wildebeest, my hearing went. Only a dull noise and a high pitched squeal came through. My mind was a blank. This was more than a five-minute spiel in front of a hand-full of people. I went to the rest room. Nothing worked there either. My body was completely shutting down. I went back outside.

Kathy was there. "You'll do just fine," she said.

With that, I walked down the auditorium aisle and onto the stage. Around me were the professors who would later become my teachers and many of them, my friends. I was literally on the stage of my life. I welcomed everyone, briefed them on the format, and introduced the next speaker.

The weekend went perfectly – except for the fact that we hadn't stocked up on toilet paper! It's always about those little details. I didn't know it then, but the event made a tremendous impression on the faculty, speakers and attendees alike and though I was exhausted, it proved to me that not only was there information to be learned about horses, there were a lot of people who wanted that knowledge.

## HER HOOF IS DEADLY ACCURATE

*Two, one-inch square holes, two inches deep appeared in the earth every time her hoof lifted off the ground. These holes now littered the earth as the pair of older men positioned the black mare for me to draw the blood for the Coggins test.*

*This blood test proved whether a horse has a communicable disease and is required in every state whenever a horse is transported, sold, or exhibited. This mare was headed to a local fair where she would be hitched to a wooden sled loaded with stones. Using the traction gained by the earth piercing cleats, she would pull the sled across a finish line. If successful, the process would be repeated with more weight until she hopefully pulled the largest load of her division and the men returned home with the purse money.*

*The only time this mare saw a vet was for the annual blood test. The men showed no interest in my inquiries about minimum vaccinations or general health. To be fair, neither did the horse. Looking at me, she made it clear she had no interest in my needle or me.*

*In preparing for my vet school licensing exam, I had measured parts of my body so I could use it as a rough measuring stick against the horse. Measured in "hands" (1 hand equals 4 inches), the tip of my nose measured 17 hands at the horse's withers. Today, as I prepared my approach to this giant, my eyes stared level into her shoulder. My eyes then looked up to see the withers that were about level with the top of my head. I was guessing her height at 19 hands when one of the men blurted at me, "Don't get too close to her Doc. She hates you already and her hoof is deadly accurate."*

*I respect every horse's potential to hurt me and pride myself in remaining calm around them. I was still about 4 feet away from her 12-inch wide hoof. She was prancing, slowly inching her body towards me. I cautiously stepped back.*

*The younger of the two old men held the shining black, overweight, and heavily muscled beast with one hand on the shank while he muttered threats directly to her. She listened and obeyed but her eyes never left mine. You could see her think.*

*The older old man grabbed a truss hammer and a loop of bailing twine. He twisted one end of the twine turning the loop into a figure 8. He folded the tips of the figure 8 together creating a circle of twine made of two loops. He repeated this twice resulting in a small circle with 8 loops of twine.*

*Next, the man slipped the head of the hammer into the middle of the circle. Grabbing 2 or 3 strands, he pulled tightly* against the hammer in the other hand drawing tight the twine against the hammer's head but exposing a few loops of twine.

"A twitch!" he said proudly. While I was amazed at this man's ingenuity, I was imagining the real trick of applying his invention to the nose of the beast.

The man holding the horse brought her to the barn wall and, standing on a stool, threaded the long rope lead through a large metal eye bolted seven feet high through the wooden frame of the barn. He firmly pulled the rope and the mare walked forward until her face was against the wall. All I could see was a disaster about to unfold including the demolition of the barn in one pull.

The mare started to show her displeasure by stomping all four hooves and shaking her head, but the other man stepped up on the stool and quickly applied the twitch. "Go ahead Doc. She's waitin' on ya."

I set my focus on the left front hoof and adjusted my stance keeping my feet in what I thought would be a safe zone. My thoughts drifted to the holes in the ground and pictured the crucifixion of my foot. I can draw blood or do an IV injection using just my right hand. Today, however, I needed my right hand to keep me away from her. I grabbed a fold of skin above the right shoulder and leaned my body into hers. She responded by leaning her full ton back on me. The twitch man growled and twisted the twitch tighter on her nose. The lead man standing on *my right side dug his thumb into her side. I raised my left hand with the sharp needle attached to a glass blood collection tube, distended her left jugular vein, and drove the needle through her thick hide. Although fine motor skills are usually a disaster with my left hand, it was a perfect stick and the blood quickly filled the tube. But my skill did not impress the lady. Her response was to start aiming her hoof. The old man yelled, "Watch it Doc. I told ya she's accurate with those feet."*

*I pulled the needle out and the men released their holds. As the mare led the men back to the stall, the oldest said, "Good job Doc!" The other said, "Yea, you're the first ever to get it done on the first try and not get hurt."*

*Smiling, I got back in my truck and waited for my knees to stop shaking and my heartbeat to end the thumping in my ears. The more horses you work with, the more your confidence builds. My respect for a horse's ability to hurt you still remains, but this day, my confidence notched a little higher.*

# CHAPTER 14

*— Now or Never —*

# CHAPTER 14

February is cold in upstate New York and cabin fever is a real mental condition brought on by continuous lack of sunshine affecting dopamine levels. I was bored to tears and in a state of limbo where I knew I would be done with my undergraduate degree in June but I had no idea what was to happen after graduation. I focused on completing the lengthy task of applying to vet school.

Part of the process included the acceptance of letters of recommendation. There was no stated limit as to the number so I sent in 14 including glowing letters from Mrs. Topper and Dr. Simpson. The following year they limited the number of letters to two and I have to wonder if maybe that was due to me.

When the weekend came along and it was between exams, Kathy and I drove about two hours north and east to Amsterdam, NY to visit her parents. Soon after arriving, Kathy's mom ushered us all into the car and we headed over to Herkimer where there was a store filled with men's suits. She was on a mission to dress me up for my interview for vet school.

I had received notice a few weeks before that I had made it to the final stage of the admission process. After the forms had been filled out and the transcripts of previous grades sent, all that was left was the interview and my mother-in-law made it her mission to wow the interviewers with a fully decked out, three piece suit that no respectable horseman would wear.

We arrived at the clothing store and I tried on suit after suit. As a rule, I don't wear suits and I was certainly not an expert. However, my mother-in-law considered herself one and she was possessed with dressing me with perfection.

A month later I was dressed in my newly tailored suit and I sat in the waiting room with other applicants who had also made it to the interview stage. We were all nervous and the constricting clothes made it worse. I had been dreaming of this moment since the notice of the interview had arrived but all I could do was feel the sweat pour from my armpits and down the sides of my vest covered shirt. I longed for the wide-open acres of the broodmare pasture way up on the top of the hill where all I could hear was the wind in the trees.

Three veterinarians were inside preparing to chew me up with questions and then spit me out upon a pile of rejections, and I'd certainly spent enough time in that pile in the past. I had little faith in a positive outcome and because of this, I developed a carefree attitude. I had convinced myself that when they asked the inevitable question, "Why do you want to become a veterinarian?" I was ready to reply, "Because no one believes a manure shoveler." I had even contemplated bringing along a bag of horse manure to emphasize my point.

We were not given instructions, just told to be there for the afternoon group. I was the last to be called in. The sweat stains on my shirt prevented me from ripping off the constricting coat, vest and tie. My heart thumped inside my chest and my body temperature rose to the point I felt half cooked. The door opened and I was ushered in.

Two vets sat on one side of a long table facing the third and I sat at the end. The silence of the room muffled my thoughts. I was on autopilot. Any rehearsed lines were gone. They smiled as I tried to recognize who they were. They were not the large animal veterinarians I had seen around the clinic as I had already attended their rounds as an uninvited undergraduate. I was sure one was a small animal vet. Oh boy, this wasn't good for me, I thought.

The questions were scripted and forgettable which made this interview seem very impersonal. I think it was an attempt to scare the crap out of people. This is a profession where a human is attached to every animal we see and if this was too much for the interviewee, then that person would not be able to handle the wrath of an irate animal owner.

My next-door neighbor, Lysanne, had a 4.04 average at Cornell (A+) and had failed her first interview because she was so nervous. I benefited though because she became my tutor in biochemistry during her wait to reapply. I'm not sure how many thrown upon the interview rejection pile had the courage to go through it again. I didn't think I would, but now, in the thick of the interview, I wasn't thinking of anything but the questions being asked.

The next question shocked me. "Geoff, we know your interest is only with horses. Tell us what you would do if that option was taken away because you became allergic to horses?" I burst into laughter, which I immediately thought was a bad idea, but it was too late. The three men stared at me with open mouths. I had already come into this interview with a carefree attitude but I had been waiting for that attitude to enter the room. With this question, I became released from my fears and allowed myself to be who I was. My burst of laughter was followed with a brief explanation that I was already allergic to them and their environmental surroundings and that I had gone through the treatment.

The interview turned around on a dime at this point. Either I felt invincible or the vets thought they were done with their charade. Either way, we broke down into a very informal hour of storytelling about everyone's experience with horses. One was impressed that I knew about the old way loose hay was plucked by grabbing claws out of hay wagons and drawn by block and tackle into the loft, then along a steel track to the back of the loft for stacking. The interview had degraded into a social gathering of like-minded people and I felt as if I was among fellow horse people, not instructors, anymore.

Unknown to me was that two very interested people had been waiting outside the interview room for my exit. Dr. Jackson and Dr. Heinrich waited as long as they could and then left. That's how long we stayed inside and talked after the 'formal' interview.

A month later, doubt set in. I had no idea what the admissions office thought of me. I only knew of my past track record and I also knew that I struggled to get a B+ average. The view I had of my application was not very good. Now, I had only one question in my mind. When I was done with this semester, what was I going to do?

Near the campus was a state forest with miles of trails. I had decided to stop worrying about school and grades. My life was about to head back to the farm. With a bachelor's degree in animal science from Cornell, I thought I would have a better salary as a farm manager. In reality, with Kathy also graduating with a bachelor's degree in farm business management, she was in a better position to get the job. Maybe I could become a truck driver. What I needed was a long walk.

Kathy and I headed out to the forest mid morning of the day that the acceptance letters were to be sent. The rain fell lightly and the low clouds touched the tops of the trees. Walking in silence I tried to put my thoughts together but it was pointless. I swung between confidence and depression. All Kathy could do was to tell me that no matter what the decision was, she loved me and all would be okay. I chose to believe her and we went home.

We had already checked the mail even though we knew it would take a day or two for the letter to get from campus to our door. Kathy started to prepare dinner as I walked pointlessly from the one room to the other and back again. The phone ringing instantly broke the strain. I answered but I became distracted as knocking came from the door at the same time.

"Hey Geoff, this is Debbie. Let me be the first to congratulate you." Debbie worked at the Equine Research Park and she always knew about everything that was going on. Before I could answer her Kathy answered the door and found our friends and vet students Mike and Chris, with a bottle of wine and huge smiles on their faces.

Debbie continued, "You got in!" My mind started to spin as relief replaced the doubt. I thanked her then turned to our guests and we celebrated for an hour. I was grateful for my friends, but I was mentally exhausted from the stress.

Kathy and I were soon alone and we chuckled like little kids. I finally fell asleep in the wee hours of the morning.

The letter arrived the next day to confirm the news. I skipped through the next few weeks, passed my exams, and went through the graduation ceremony. I felt like I had accomplished my goal of entering vet school. I had yet to realize that getting in was the easiest part.

I worked all summer at the Equine Research Park and my status with Dr. Jackson rose from undergraduate to first year vet student with all the responsibilities associated with it. The excitement continued to grow as welcoming packages arrived and the orientation schedule became firm.

The day all the new students came together, we were in the cafeteria. The dean of admissions asked us to stand up and introduce ourselves. The familiar panic set in as I listened and watched everyone stand up and say something about themselves. They all seemed confident and intelligent and young. It was my turn and I said something but I only heard my own name. After we were all done, I couldn't remember anyone's name or anything about them. I felt a little lost and in way over my head.

I wondered for a while why I had been placed last on the list to be interviewed that day. The answer came several years later after I had become friends with the secretary of the dean of Admissions.

It was three years into my veterinary education when she and I were talking. I was reminiscing about my interview day as I saw her working on that year's applicant files. When I told her how nervous I had been she laughed out loud. She exclaimed, "You were nervous? Why? You were the school's number one pick."

## MY TURN TO TRIM THE TOES

*There was a brief time when I worked for another practice and honestly, the boss and I didn't get along. One of the favorite things he would do was to send employees he didn't like out to do things that were not in the scope of being an equine practitioner.*

*It was a hot summer day in upstate New York and in the lazy afternoon heat of the practice vehicle I had fallen asleep. That was okay because I was 30 minutes early for the appointment I had been assigned. The snickers from my fellow employees had not distracted me from what had looked like an easy afternoon.*

*I was in such a deep sleep that I could have been in another world. I had parked across the street from a two story red brick colonial house in an upscale community. There was no evidence of any farming. Not even a vegetable patch let alone a fence for animals. I had been asked to trim the toes of a pot-bellied pig and I had checked the address several times to be sure I was in the right place.*

*The owner arrived from work in the city and surprised me as she woke me from my depths of sleep with a smart wave and brilliant smile from across the street. She was dressed in a bright red patterned skirt, a white fluffy blouse, legs enhanced with stockings, and smooth black high heels. Sparkling jewelry accented her arms and neck and her hair and makeup had not weathered from her day at the office. She did not look like the usual "barn girl" I see every day.*

*I entered the house that was spotless. She turned to me and said, "Don't let him know you are here to trim his feet. He will squeal and run. I can't even trim my nails in front of him."*

*I was dressed in green coveralls and somewhat clean work boots. I grasped a pair of hoof nippers and a rasp in one hand and raised the other in an open palm of assurance and said, "No problem! Where is the little pig, outside?"*

*She acted a little surprised with my question and then said that he was in the living room. "It is his favorite spot to lay between the couch and coffee table." I entered the room with the thoughts of quickly getting this job done and continuing with my day.*

*There was not a speck of dirt anywhere in the well-appointed room with wall-to-wall white carpeting and a white couch in an L shape. Small items were spread over the large coffee table. I approached from the back of the couch sticking out into the room. As I peered over the top of it, I quickly began to reassess* the situation. I yelped, "I thought you had a small pot bellied pig!" Snoring and filling all space available was a 400-pound sleeping pig! The lady looked at me with a look of assurance for I was the hero who had come to rescue her beastly friend from long hooves. The snickers back at the office came ringing through my thoughts as I attempted to develop a new plan.

With the same empty feeling of jumping out of a plane to parachute for the first time, I launched my body on top of the sleeping monster and grabbed the nearest leg and started snipping excess hoof. The squeal cut through my soul and split my eardrums. The pig legs flailed as the couch escaped the scene.

The first cloven hoof was done at least to my specifications anyway, which at that point was somewhat less than what we would expect from a trained journeyman farrier. The pig was really rocking at this point and for a moment it looked like I might be done with this fight. I was now sprawled with my chest and stomach on top of the pig as I waited for the eight-second buzzer.

The woman who had been speechless and watching up to this point came to my rescue and threw herself on top of me. The pig increased his squealing. For a moment, my thoughts went somewhere else as the woman's body embraced the pig and me. But as a professional, I knew I had been given the advantage over the pig for a few moments and I grabbed the other forelimb. While the three of us became intimate, I nipped off the excess hoof material. A moment later the woman and I were tossed aside in a pile as the pig made his escape squealing for his life.

*We picked each other up and straightened out our clothes. For a moment there was silence as my heart pounded. Then without any warning, the kitchen door opened and her husband burst through and said, "Ya need any help out here?"*

# CHAPTER 15

*— Dr. Tucker —*

# CHAPTER 15

The first two years were a blur from the constant workload. Added to this was my mom visiting us one day with an offer to buy some start up land for a farm. At first it didn't make any sense to purchase land in Ithaca. I had always set my sights on Kentucky, but my fate was sealed when we became the owners of 100 acres of land in Freeville, NY about 14 miles from the university.

The house that came with the property was disgusting and that was on its best day! Asphalt shingles on the roof along with thick cardboard for siding made this structure an eyesore. The former owner lived in a small modular home next door and on the other side of the house was a mobile home. The back yard was scrub brush with deer paths I would use to walk the dogs at night.

Mill Creek flowed across the property dividing the front ten acres with the house from the remaining property. It could be crossed during the dry season and I loved walking the dogs in the back woods. This was a time when I could get away from the classes and stress. That was not often as vet school consumed almost every hour of my life starting with early morning rounds.

Rounds are when a veterinary department offers 30 to 60 minutes of case presentations and students sit or stand as the clinician works a case up and then brings the affected animal for all to see. The first time I had heard of rounds was when my grandfather had his hip replaced back in 1970. Because he was one of the first to have this done, he was wheeled out onto the auditorium stage in his wheelchair as the surgeons who had just performed the operation asked him questions. I smiled each time an animal was brought out before the crowd of students as I thought of how proud my grandfather was when he was in his spotlight.

My first set of rounds was called Postmortem Rounds and was held every Friday afternoon at 4:30. I entered the postmortem presenting room divided from the abattoir by swinging stainless steel doors. Everything within the glazed brick room was made of stainless steel with a large floor drain. Cleaning was done with hosing and disinfectant.

In the middle of the room were two or three steel tables each with a hole off to the side so blood and fluids could drain to the bucket hanging below the hole. Circled around the tables were five sets of grandstand seating also made of stainless steel. The seating was tight and we all angled our knees so they would not press into the backs of the people seated in front of us. I always went for the top row to see better, though the lowest seat was the closest.

At exactly 4:30, the chief pathologist would enter the room and command attention. His eyes remained focused on the specimens laying on the tables that the assistants had selected for rounds. Hearts, lungs, livers, bladders, heads, and every other part you could think of were presented. The chief with rubber gloves and a rubber apron would pick up with one hand the discolored liver with pus nodules and fibrin tags evident on its surface and with the other hand, take the worlds sharpest knife and make several slices into the organ. "Diagnosis?" he would say in a large voice.

A student would give an answer, then be sucked into a series of more questions such as, "Species?" or "Cause?" or "Wrong!" Only the confident would open their mouths. I, being only an undergraduate at first then later an infant vet student sitting in the back row, kept my lips firmly pressed together. My eyes remained wide open as I became fascinated with the damage a disease would cause. By the time I had entered vet school, the chief recognized me often bringing his eyes to meet mine daring me to open my mouth. I rarely did because of the other smarter upperclassmen there. I did, however, answer his questions silently to myself and became proud when I knew the answer.

Other rounds included Large Animal, Small Animal, Lameness (horses), Ophthalmology, and Neurology Rounds. We would watch the clinicians and hear their stories about the case while we students would sip coffee and eat our breakfast bagel in the pre-school hours. The time always flew by and we would flee to our 8 am class entering a few minutes late. For me, Rounds were the best part of my veterinary education.

Our introduction to the use of drugs started with the new head of the pharmacology department standing up in front of the class and announcing the syllabus of the semester that included land cultivation, crop rotation, etc. We were all confused until the professor stopped and apologized saying he thought this was the "farm ecology" course.

I use goofy comedy all the time, but this really bothered me. Attending veterinary school was in my mind a serious exercise and for the head of the department to joke seemed foreign. As time went on I began to realize that comedy and humor does play an important part in everything we do. Bringing perspective to life, the landmarks humor brings to an otherwise barren landscape allows for good memories. It also made all the hard work bearable.

Dr. Forrester was our instructor in large animal medicine. He had been practicing since the first veterinary license had been granted and probably 100 years before that. Wisdom clearly exemplified his knowledge and his way of teaching us was a mix of facts and stories. He carried his loose-leaf notebook into class, found his place from the last lecture, and start in exactly where he had left off from the previous class. He was in automatic mode as he recited what he knew about lung or kidney disease in cows, horses, pigs, and small ruminants. Often his eyes would close and I often thought there was a tape recorder playing as he stood motionless before us.

His delivery was slow enough for me to sleep well during class, but his stories always had me and my classmates wide awake. My dilemma of afternoon naps during his lectures needed a plan. Two solutions came to me. The first was from my classmate Josh who often brought me a bag of corn nuts. I would suck on the salty fried corn kernel until it was semisoft, and then crack the rest between my teeth. If performed too early, the sound would disturb my neighbors. Too late and it would not have the snap necessary to keep me awake.

My other solution was to transcribe his lectures. Years later I would read my notes from his class and it was like an audio recording with every nuance and tone inflection perfectly preserved. This busy work kept me awake.

I was sad to end his class as the semester drew to an end, but his famous final oral exam was worth the wait because I thoroughly enjoyed oral exams. With my learning difficulties, written exams only confused me. Oral exams on the other hand gave me a stage where thoughts and ideas could flow into my head easily. A question would be asked and I would start my answer. As words flowed from my mouth, a floodgate would open into my mind's "assembly room" and in mid sentence, I could change direction, which was usually good when I was on the wrong track.

Our class assembled into the large room as Dr. Forrester remained in his office. A list was handed out which gave the order as well as the three person groups that were to enter his office. I was grouped with two other ladies who were interested in small animals only.

I sat listening to everyone's nervous chatter. Most of them were about to pee in their pants and had already assumed their career was over. The thought of taking an oral exam was their worst fear. The energy was peaking and I couldn't take it anymore. I went over to the two nervous girls scheduled to take the oral exam with me. "Hey!" I exclaimed. "What are you fretting for? You all know this stuff. In another year all we will have our oral exams on a daily basis."

"What are you talking about?" one asked.

I quickly remembered that I was five years older and had more experience in the real world. I tried to relate to them that every day clients would be asking us questions about their animals and that Dr. Forrester was only doing just that, asking questions about an animal. If we couldn't face a colleague, how on earth would we be able to face a client? The women's faces looked back with a complete lack of understanding.

At least I tried, but I saw this reaction often with my classmates. The three of us were called into Dr. Forrester's cramped office stuffed with his big body, three extra chairs, and hundreds of items collected over the years from his practice with large animals. He looked at us through his thick glasses and summed up the students before him. I was silent but the two girls twitched and sputtered words. Dr. Forrester smiled as he saw his victims squirm before their death. The sweat started to drip from my armpits as I became aware of my own nervousness.

He turned to me first. "Doc? What... in the name of God..............is this?" The words were drawn out for emphasis and his high-pitched voice squeaked out of his nasal caverns. I was handed an object made of dried cow manure about six inches long. It had a tube shape about two inches in diameter with a one-inch hole running through the middle of it.

As I have said, I love oral exams because of the way my mind works. In a written exam, I am given a limited amount of words to work with but when I visualize something, my mind opens up to a thousand times the possibilities for answers. In today's terms, it is the difference between two computers, one with ten times the memory.

A flood of possibilities flashed in my mind and in an instant, I started a discussion about calf scours. Bang! I had nailed it. He asked a few more questions about it and I was done. All the studying about all the diseases and everything was over on a question on calf diarrhea. I don't remember the questions to the girls. I did know that I was going to pass large animal medicine and that there was nothing that would stop me from graduating. However, the school knew there was one more lesson to be taught. It was the art of working with people.

We were not ready for the public so most of our class work was done on animals owned by the school. The thought of standing in front of a real client frightened most of us and the school knew it. To overcome this, the school set up vaccination clinics throughout the county for dogs and cats.

I have to say I would rather die than work on small animals. This was generally the opposite opinion of my classmates who looked forward to donning the white lab coat and grabbing "Precious" by the scurf of the flabby neck and stabbing the needle under the skin. I did my best work in blue jeans, a flannel shirt, and work boots. Standing next to a half-ton beast quicker than a striking snake made me feel at home. One hiss and growl from one of those fanged mini tigers and I knew I would bail and run.

I had no experience with dogs and cats other than in my childhood when my cat was run over by a car and killed and my dog was stolen for research. My current dog, E-Z, I considered to be part human and didn't count as a dog in my opinion. When my assigned Saturday arrived, I drove to the local firehouse of a town as far away from where I lived as I could select. I wore a pair of khaki pants, an oxford shirt and tie, and the obligatory white coat. I really looked the part but I sure didn't feel it.

The line of town folk formed outside the firehouse eager to get their balls of fur vaccinated for free. Four of my classmates and I huddled around the young clinician assigned to watch over us and guide us through what I thought surely would be a nightmare.

The vet in charge and I took a position by a table set up in the garage where the fire trucks usually parked. The familiar cold sweat dripped down my armpits and my breathing became shallow as the first man brought his slightly overweight mixed breed dog up to the table. I let him sniff my hand as I squelched every nerve of anxiety from my mind.

Acting as if I had done this a million times, I took the protective cap off the needle, lifted the tail of the dog straight up in the air like it was a 1500 pound stallion, and drove the needle deep into his hind leg muscle. As the poor dog cried out with a sharp yelp of irritation with me, I simultaneously injected the liquid into the beast and turned away quickly as if this dog's reaction was normal.

"Thanks!" I said followed by, "Next!" My heart was pounding in my chest and I was hyperventilating. I envisioned the dog having a seizure from my restraint technique and the inadvertent injection of the substance directly into an artery. The room started to spin as I suddenly realized that the injection should have gone under the skin, not in the leg muscle like a horse!

Out of the corner of my eye I saw the dog licking the man's face madly as he pet his head. I imagined him saying, "Oh, did that mean Doctor hurt you? Well, with the money I saved today, I'm going get you a biscuit." The dog's tail wagged and they both headed out the door.

I was feeling relieved that I might make it through the day, but my hopes quickly vanished as I turned to see a young lady place her cat, who was in a cat container, on the table. I panicked. There was no way I was going to reach inside that cave and extract that crazed fanged monster with razor sharp talons.

I looked for help and saw my classmates smiling and even laughing as happy people lined up at their stations looking genuinely excited to be part of this initiation of veterinary plebes. Thankfully, the instructor saw me and came over.

"How are you doing?" he asked with the calmness of an angel.

"Fine!" I lied.

"Well, who do we have here?" he asked of the young girl as he slowly opened up the cage door. His hands gently reached in and lifted the purring cat out.

I heard a high pitched ringing in my ears as the blood pumping at twice it's normal pressure seared over my ear drums. I could barely hear anything as my inner voice kept trying to calm me down. Then, as clear as on a quiet morning, he said, "Dr. Tucker, are you ready?"

It was the first time anyone had called me "Dr. Tucker" in public. Even though I was technically not a doctor yet, the words transformed me. Time stood still as I suddenly realized that this was it. I was "over the hump." There was no going back and this wasn't a dream.

Against all odds I had made it through the ranks. The next 12 months would be a breeze. My veins filled with confidence I never realized I had. The impact of that one teacher was so profound on my future it cannot be measured. I picked up the syringe and quickly inserted it under the skin and injected the vaccine. The cat purred without a hiccup.

The rest of the day went so smoothly I couldn't wait to get home to tell Kathy. Dr. Tucker was home for dinner.

# A Case Of Walking Pneumonia

*The autumn weather in upstate New York can be glorious and this day was perfect in every way. My call that day was to examine an unthrifty horse. Looking at him in his pasture run in shed, I knew something wasn't right but finding the cause was proving difficult. Back then, running blood tests was a lengthy thing to do and veterinarians needed to look harder for answers using more skills than just technology.*

*I held the big gelding's nostrils closed until he started to fight for air. Releasing my grasp of his nose, he gratefully drew in a large and deep breath. My stethoscope pressed close to his chest as I strained to hear abnormal lung sounds. I was rewarded with a very faint squeak. "Pneumonia!" I triumphantly said to the man holding the horse as the excitement for my detective skills escaped with my report to the owner of the horse. "Your horse has a case of walking pneumonia," I continued to explain.*

*The owner quickly asked, "How did he get that and what do I do for it?"*

*After explaining this case the best I could to the owner, I prescribed a powerful antibiotic along with instructions on how to give the intravenous injection. Everything seemed good with the man as my truck tires found the black top of the road and I headed to the next farm. Satisfaction with my diagnosis and confidence in the treatment allowed me to tell the owner that his horse should be okay. It was textbook routine, so I went on my way and didn't give it another thought.*

*Reexamination of the horse took place five days later. The tone of the farm was somber. I worried that the horse was not responding to the treatment. Instead of feeling good, I felt a pervasive coldness on the whole property.*

The owner's wife haltered the horse and presented him to me. He appeared bright and alert and his hair coat had recovered its luster. I listened to the lungs and they sounded much better. I was relieved. All seemed right as I announced the good news, but my positive attitude had no effect, as the woman was distant. I asked her if everything was all right.

"No," she said. "My husband was upset after you left last week, after your diagnosis of pneumonia in the horse." She paused and I wondered if he was upset with me or with the disease.

She then said, "My husband was a disturbed man but he loved his horse. Two days after you left, he sat in his favorite chair in our living room and blew his brains out."

I was speechless. The news shook me to the core, blanking my mind into emptiness. It changed my life as a veterinarian forever.

Her anger with his actions was evident and I let her speak. I was now treating the owner and not the horse.

From that day on I realized that veterinarians are not just treating the animal. We are treating the owner through their animal. I have worked hard to make my visits a happy event where the owner feels like they have been heard.

I certainly don't feel responsible for that man's death but knowing I was part of his life's script, even in a minor role, makes me careful not to tip another life over their edge.

# CHAPTER 16

*— The Value of a Life —*

# CHAPTER 16

The editor of *The Blood Horse* magazine had come to offer a scholarship to help veterinary students become better equine veterinarians. His thought was that the students needed more real world experience before coming out of school. He sat down with me and two other classmates, all of us personally chosen by the administration and all interested in working with horses after graduation.

My experience of "out in the real world" was vast compared to Mary and Pat who sat to my left. The editor laid out his proposition offering money to two deserving 3rd year vet students. He asked us what would be a good amount to offer. My classmates came up with $200.

"What?" I blurted. "$200? Have you paid any bills lately?" I asked. The man eyed me with interest. I continued, "I'm married and have living expenses for two plus tuition and school costs. I think $2000 is more reasonable."

I gulped as silence embraced the moment. I knew, however, that anything less would be a waste of my time. Allowing a student the opportunity to work for an established equine practice and glean all the experience of the clinicians without compensating those of us working through college automatically prejudiced us from those whose bills were being paid by someone else. As my logic settled in, I realized that my classmates did not understand that Kathy and I had no outside financial help and we were actually working to pay the bills and working to graduate.

The editor instantly understood me and said he would match up to $2000 if the employer would hire the student for $2000 in summer employment. I was elated with this and we all floated out of the room. A month later the scholarship was announced and I was one of the two accepted into the program. I was very excited.

When the summer of 1983 came around, I had secured employment with an equine practice in the Hudson Valley of New York. I drove to work on Monday leaving my farm in Freeville at 4:30 in the morning and arrived at the practice just before 8 am. During the week I slept in the guest bedroom of Arlene who was the bookkeeper of the practice.

Every morning I awoke quietly leaving the house and drove to a local Thoroughbred training facility arriving at 6:30 am. The farm was in full swing at that hour and I headed out to locate the manager. My bosses had arranged for me to float the teeth of all the horses in training after they realized my interest in horse teeth. Every morning I would work on two or three two year olds before driving to the clinic.

How good was my work? Not very good compared to what I do now but I learned so much about wolf teeth and caps. These horses weren't the easiest to work with either and I received a fair share of bruises and cuts. I also worked up a good appetite. I looked forward to pulling over for food on the way to the first call, which was usually a buttered hard roll and soda.

Most of my time was split between Dr. Ronson, the senior partner, and Dr. Proll who is still working at the practice today. Dr. Ronson took me under his wing and became an incredible mentor. This man always worked, and always drank. We drove mostly to dairy farms but we also did a fair share of horse work. At night we would return to his farm and I would help him bale hay. I was one of the stackers placing the bales as they came off the kicker into the following wagon. I would then stack the bales into his loft. The beer would flow and the laughter became constant. He impressed upon me the need to keep life simple.

Dr. Proll became my horse mentor that summer and for him I am eternally grateful. Like Dr. Ronson, he also believed in keeping life light, but he was also capable of becoming serious when needed. His life lessons remain with me today. A habit he started with me was to allow the clients to call him any name they felt comfortable with. Doctor Proll, Doc, and first name - anything they wanted was okay with him. Another habit was to place a block of wood on his dash. Every day, somewhere in a conversation, he would reach over and tap the wood with his knuckles and say, "Knock on wood." Today, I have a Staple's "That Was Easy" button on my dash and I use it in the same way.

During the evenings after calls, Dr. Proll had projects for me on his farm that helped supplement my cash. He learned of my unending ability to work. For this he reciprocated with an unending desire to teach. I received the better part of the deal.

One day Dr. Proll had in his mind he was going to learn how to place medication into a horse's hock using a needle. In 1983, no one was doing this except a handful of university professors. Before I had left Cornell, a new resident that year was experimenting with the procedure. Today every vet student has performed joint injections routinely, but on this summer's day, Dr. Proll had set his jaw in determination.

The client Dr. Proll had selected to ask was very willing to have his horse experimented on. He had found a how-to article and used my fresh student experience to analyze it. "Geoffrey," he always called me by my full first name, "today we are going to learn how to do this thing."

We arrived and as we got out of his truck, Dr. Proll reached up and knocked his block of wood. He anesthetized the horse and while the animal lay motionless on the ground, he and I became equal in learning. We poked and prodded until we were certain of the location. In went the needle and out came the joint fluid. Dr. Proll was as happy as he could be. No "new thing" was going to leave him behind, not if it made sense to him.

The horse recovered nicely and no harm was done. While this was a great learning experience for both of us, Dr. Proll's greatest gift was for recognizing things as they were. "If it walks like a duck and quacks like a duck, it's a duck" was one of his favorite expressions. I have never thought like that because my imagination allows me to overanalyze everything. His simplicity amazed me and helped me to calm my brain as I learned to think through critical events.

The summer was important to me because it joined my experience on the farm with the new knowledge I was learning in vet school. My confidence working as an equine vet exponentially increased as I became aware of the simplicity of it. An example of this came one afternoon at one of the Dream Street dairy farms scattered throughout Westchester and Putnam Counties of New York. The principal owner of the farms was Yoko Ono, the widow of John Lennon. These Holstein cows were the best in the country, if not the world. They lived in cleanliness unsurpassed by most people's living room standards.

Dr. Ronson took me to a case of milk fever there. The large black and white cow was putting all of her blood calcium into her udder for milk. This weakens the cow causing many symptoms including her inability to stand. She was curled up on her chest in the thickly bedded stall filled with golden wheat straw. I had brought in all the equipment and supplies necessary to get her back on her feet. I had been to many of these cases before with him.

"Okay, get her head Geoff," Dr. Ronson confidently said to me. I placed the rope halter over her head and tied it without resistance back to her side curving the outer side of her neck. The large jugular vein could easily be seen slowly pulsing under the skin.

Dr. Ronson just looked at me, then with a slight smile and a glint in his eye, said, "All right, get that needle in and hook her up."

I blinked for a moment but knew we were standing in front of the barn owner. In my best effort to not shake the confidence of the herd boss, I immediately took the needle and drove it deep into her blood pipe. It was a perfect stick and I quickly hooked up the line and started to run the calcium fluids into her body.

Dr. Ronson looked pleased with how things had turned out. I settled in for the ten-minute administration of the medicine. Calcium works very quickly when given intravenously but there is a consideration to how fast it is administered. Too fast and the cow's heart can develop an arrhythmia and stop. I used my stethoscope listening to the gurgle of fresh fluid enter her heart. If I noticed the rate or rhythm of the heart change, I would drop the bottle lower to the ground and this would slow the administration. Too low and her blood would back up into the tube which indicated the administration rate was zero.

I was in autopilot mode. It must have showed because Dr. Ronson suddenly broke from his conversation with the barn owner to ask me how I was doing.

I said, "Fine."

Then he asked me, "Does it ever bother you when you know the value of the animal?"

I answered, "Nope, it makes no difference."

"Good!" he exclaimed, "Cause this cow is worth $100,000."

My arm was extended above my body as far as it could go holding the bottle and the fluids were pouring into the cow rapidly. As the words "One Hundred Thousand Dollars" settled into the reading room of my mind, the sweat pores in my armpits opened up and my side became soaked. My arm reflexively dropped and my attention focused on her heart. All was good.

I wanted to argue with myself that I really believed the cost of the animal really did not make a difference. However,

I became plagued with the idea that the higher the value of the animal, the higher I needed to perform. What happened that afternoon with Dr. Ronson and the Dream Street cow soon became profound in my practice life. I settled my argument decisively and settled on the idea that the value in dollars is a man made idea. The value of life is equal and is only determined by the individual. Dr. Ronson knew this when he asked me to work on this expensive animal. He had noticed my complacency and needed to correct it, which he did perfectly. He would have done the same on a two-dollar cow.

It's easy sometimes to forget how connected someone may be to an animal and though in the case of a dairy farm, cows are largely considered numbers, it's rarely that way with most of the animals I treat. Sometimes, especially when I was younger, I didn't really understand that things that were more or less routine for me weren't always so routine for the owners.

# WHAT CORNELL FORGOT TO TEACH ME

*Spending almost every waking hour of my life over four years learning veterinary medicine made me the most intelligent horse expert walking the planet upon graduation. I had learned every part of the horse's body, every disease they could contract, every part of the breeding cycle, and every foaling event that could occur. Nutrition and husbandry for horses including parasite control and vaccination protocols were deeply embedded in my abundantly trained mind. I was as prepared as a vet could be to walk into the cold cruel world of animals and become the hero.*

*Of course there were ccountless cases in my first year that made me realize I had not learned everything and there would be years of "practice" before I would feel confident in my veterinary skills. Here are two stories describing my sobering experiences in a mixed animal practice within my first year of my veterinary career. One is with a horse and another with a cow.*

## USED MOTOR OIL

*The horse farm in this rural area wasn't really a farm. It was a small run down dairy farm that at first glance looked more like a junkyard. The long dirt driveway cut back sharply from the main road and descended slowly through woods and brush before spreading into a wide-open lot filled with discarded and decaying farm equipment. "Blue Angel" silos belonging to financially productive dairy farms were absent from this squandered dairy farm. Their monies had been unwisely spent on barely get-by equipment and repairs rather than professionally equipped barns and implements.*

*I parked my truck near a cluttered corral made of repaired boards surrounding cement and dirt. Within its' confines were scattered hay, a water pail, and a small black horse who was my patient.*

*"Doc, as I told your office, this colt has a skin condition," the owner said gruffly. "We've been treating him for a while but it ain't working, so we called you. What do you think?"*

*I stared at this horse in poor condition that was covered from his nose to his tail with a black oily substance. He sadly stood for my examination, which was brief. My fingers touched the matted hair and slid on the medication the owner had applied. The odor I was familiar with from my days working on cars.*

*"What is this?" I asked.*

*"It's a good coating of used motor oil," he proudly replied.*

*I searched my brain for the lecture where they taught me about this skin treatment but quickly realized Cornell had skipped over it.*

*It was bath time for this horse. Even though the soap would remove the oil and medication would heal the skin, the horse remained with people who had created the poor living conditions as well as the caustic treatment. Cornell had forgotten to mention that to me as well.*

## AN EVENING C-SECTION

*I was a horse vet on emergency night duty in a primarily dairy practice and I was only a few months out of vet school. The call caught me just before heading to bed, which is far better than after sliding under the fresh sheets and drifting off to the first deep part of rejuvenating sleep. It was a cow having problems delivering her calf.*

*Most dairy farms are different from horse farms in one fundamental way. The cows are treated in a more business like manor with emotions usually being left for things like family. When I arrived the barn owner met me and brought me to the cow in question. I cleaned her up and entered her birth canal discovering a very large calf stuck in the narrow hipbones of the heifer. I reported my findings to the man who basically excused himself to go off to bed wishing me good luck as he disappeared into the milk house.*

*The only approach to this was to do a Cesarean Section and deliver the calf through a hole I would cut in her side. I started to look seriously at the facts. I was sure this was a two-man job and I was the only one in the barn. It was also the first C-section I had ever done.*

*I called Doug, my boss. It was about 10 at night and he was in bed asleep. He gets up to go to his own dairy barn for chores by 4. "Doug, I have a C-section to do and I could use some help," I said hoping not to sound like I was pleading.*

*"Geoff," he replied with a sound of annoyance, "you will have no problem with this." With a click, he hung up.*

*I stood there alone in the dimly lit barn, 30 other cows quietly stood munching their evening hay, and the smell of fresh fetal fluids wafted from half way down the barn.*

*I entered the depths of my training memories and went through what I needed to do, returned to the truck to get the extra supplies, and buckled down to work. An hour later I was struggling to lower a 150-pound bull calf from the hole in the cow's side to the ground. I dragged it forward to the curious heifer and she licked it as I sutured the uterus and then the abdominal wall and skin.*

*Returning home exhausted, physically and mentally drained, I reflected again on what Cornell had forgotten to teach me. They forgot to tell me that there would be no one to hold my hand in the real world when things became tough. In one short sentence, my new boss had taught me to dig down deep and find within me what was necessary to get things done when I was telling myself it was impossible.*

# CHAPTER 17

*— A Healing Connection —*

# CHAPTER 17

Education's number one goal, I believe, is to teach one to think. Anyone can learn facts and figures, but to get out of tough situations, it is required to use one's brain.

One example came on an evening where, as a senior vet student, I was on call for small animal emergencies. The frantic owners of the mixed breed dog had a look of panic on their faces. Their dog had been given a 1-inch thick section of a cow's leg bone to chew on. These are round circles of bone with an empty hole in the center where the marrow had been.

This dog had slipped the bone over his lower jaw and it had become trapped behind his large two lower canine teeth. I examined the dog and gave the brilliant diagnosis of a bone being stuck on this dog's jaw. But I became stumped on just how to remove the bone. It was time to call for some help.

Andy was the small animal resident on call that night and who I was assigned to work with. Graduating from Cornell a year ahead of me, he was a tall, skinny comedian who turned everything into a joke. I thought he was a little less than the ideal person I wanted to save this animal from years of suffering. The owners on the other hand took one look at the confident man clad in white from top to bottom and they immediately showed relief. My ability to present myself as the person to save the day for this dog never materialized as I was stumped.

These owners were nearly sobbing tears as they saw the sad look of helplessness in their dog's eyes. But Andy's presence calmed everyone and even the dog wagged his tail and offered no resistance to his attempts at removal. However, nothing worked and soon the atmosphere became a little shaky. The next step to keep the owners calm was to remove the dog from view while we continued to try and figure things out.

Once in the back, Andy's true personality began to shine as his panic set in. "What the heck do we do now?" he said as profanity spewed from his mouth. I offered the suggestion of a bone saw and Andy ordered, "Run to the postmortem room and get theirs." I soon returned and with the dog sedated, we cut the cow bone off of the jaw.

Everyone was happy except the clinician in charge who said something about disease from the PM room possibly transferring into the clinics. Maybe so, but I learned that improvising is good.

I also learned in the small animal clinics that technique trumped force. I would never think to out muscle a thousand pound horse, but somehow when I had to deal with small animals, force seemed like the only way to escape injury. My classmate Tim and I were trying to take blood from a cat's jugular vein once. The cat weighed maybe two pounds at most. We were both big, strong men and we thought that this would be a simple 3 second procedure. The cat thought otherwise.

I laid the cat on the stainless steel table and positioned her toward the edge. I wrapped my arms around the cat in the way I had been instructed trapping the body and all legs from reaching out to scratch us. With one hand I extended the head upwards to expose the jugular vein and Tim proceeded to perform the stick.

It was a disaster. The needle went flying and I barely escaped my own massive blood loss. We regrouped. Now Tim was holding the cat using the same technique. I carefully wiped down the fur over the jugular with alcohol to help the vein stand out. I aimed and drove the needle into the skin.

Again, fur flew everywhere and hissing sounds with gurgles and growls a tiger would be proud of emanated from this small, sweet little kitty. Tim's glasses were half off his face. We were regrouping once again when Dr. Carter, the head of small animal medicine, entered the exam room to find out what the fuss was.

She looked at us and asked, "What are you big fellows trying to do here?"

We stammered, "We are trying to get a blood sample."

"So what's the problem?" she asked.

We started to collect the cat but this time the linebackers were going to immobilize that furry two-pound monster.

"Stop," Dr. Carter said. She put her things down and said to us, "Step back." She calmly stroked the head of the cat and said soothing words. Then, without any effort to control the beast and by herself, she smoothly slipped the needle into the vein and extracted the blood into the glass tube.

All Tim and I could do was watch with our mouths open. She turned to us with the vial of blood in one hand and the purring cat in the other arm, smiled and said, "Guys, it's technique, not strength." Words I live by to this day.

My final story from the small animal clinic comes from my own cat, Tinka. A car in front of my house hit her and I had brought her into the clinic. She had been knocked and rolled but no bones were broken. I was grateful and the clinicians gave approval for her return to my house that night.

I placed her on our bed and I watched her the rest of the day, but she didn't move. She had no desire to eat or drink and I didn't have to be a vet student to understand that something was wrong. I went for the thermometer and stethoscope. I inserted the thermometer into the rectum and began listening to the heart and lungs. After a minute I checked the temperature. I thought I had forgotten to shake down the mercury. I shook it down to below 96 and reinserted it then waited. I watched as the mercury climbed past 100, 102, 104, and finally stopped when there was no more room for expansion at 106. I bundled her up in a towel and returned to the clinic.

The surgical resident on duty that night was another angel named Dr. Thompson. She had a calming aura that set me at ease. She took one look and declared, "Time to operate." I was confused. I was looking at a cat with a very high fever but no reason to operate.

Dr. Thompson was as tall as me and together we hovered over Tinka now anesthetized and laying on her back. The prep had happened very fast. The belly was shaved by one tech while the anesthetist had passed the trachea tube and hooked up the gas machine. Before I knew it, Tinka's abdomen was cut open and her intestines were exposed.

It was not what I had expected to see. It looked more like someone had thrown in their three day old trash into her belly. Then, before I could blink, Dr. Thompson started to pour several liters of chilled saline directly into the mess of intestines. As she did this, she turned to me and said, "This is the quickest way to lower a fever that high!"

Her brilliance was obvious yet as my mind reviewed all the classes I attended, it became apparent that this obvious approach had been missed. It was a good lesson that some things are urgent and don't make sense and when that happens you have to get in there and look round. Waiting for blood analysis or evaluation with high tech machines wasn't needed. Just cold fluids in the abdomen and as an added benefit, we were able to see that the pancreas had been injured by the car's impact. The digestive juices normally contained within the digestive tract had leaked out and were digesting Tinka's internal organs. Dr. Thompson quickly cleaned things up and sent my cat to the Intensive Care Unit.

Katie was the vet technician during the day and in charge of everything. Vets never questioned her and she never overstepped her bounds. She became a keen observer of things as she worked tirelessly for years in the small animal clinic. After about a week of my visits to Tinka during my lunch break, Katie stopped me. "Geoff, your cat just sleeps all morning. When the vets or students come to do their exam of her she acts lifeless. Then you come for lunch and she lights up and becomes alive again. She stays that way for an hour or so after you leave. It is truly remarkable. Maybe we should allow all owners visiting rights."

She was right. Her response to my visits was easily seen by anyone watching and showed clearly the bond between owner and animal. I have used this throughout my career allowing the owner to hang out and visit anytime I worked on their animals. There were exceptions to this. Over the years I've asked owners to leave when they start to freak out and make the horse nervous. Usually, though, the opposite occurs. There is a connection between all owners and their animals and that connection has the power to heal, I'm convinced of it. Though it may never appear as a fact in a medical text anywhere, I have seen and experienced it for myself so many times that I know it's true.

I need to add a note here about small animals and me. While I have mentioned several times that I hate to work on dogs and cats, I need to be clear that I have owned numerous dogs and cats throughout my life and have loved all of them. More importantly, throughout my training at Cornell, I can say that I learned more about thinking like a doctor from my small animal instructors and animal handlers. Every one of them had an enormous impact on the development of the veterinarian I am today and my gratefulness cannot be adequately measured.

# THE SHAVE CREAM DELIVERY

*The 911 page came as I stood in front of the mirror, my razor poised over my face covered in thick, white cream. It was just past six in the morning and my automated morning rituals were in jeopardy of being cast aside by this emergency. Kathy was on foaling duty all night in our barn and I was on my own this morning with additional responsibilities of waking my son and getting him going.*

*Cell phones had not been developed yet and the method of communication at the time was an answering service and a pager. The horse owner would call Sue or Diane at the message center, they would tell them what was going on, and then a page would be sent to me alerting me to an important message.*

*My wife also had the number to my pager. This morning's page was urgent from my wife. She was in the barn and I ran out only in my pants, boots, and shave cream.*

*The mare had just started foaling and there were only two hooves showing. I saw immediately that things were not right. Normally when a foal is delivered, the two front hooves present with the soles facing down followed by the nose of the foal. What struck me odd was that both hooves had their soles facing up.*

*My truck was parked next to the barn. I ignored the cold spring air against my bare chest as I opened doors and pulled out my foaling equipment. I didn't need much. I knew this was* a simple posterior presentation. In other words, the foal was coming out back end first.

I washed up the mare and my arms and lubricated everything and then I dove in to explore and confirm that the presentation was as I thought. The mare elected to remain standing. I grabbed both hind legs of the foal and gently but firmly pulled as the mare pushed the foal's large hips through her birth canal. Twisting the foal along with rocking it side to side, I encouraged the mare to try again. She gave a big push and the foal burst free. I caught the limp and slimy mass in my arms and guided it to a soft landing onto the clean bedding. Total time was about 10 minutes.

I looked to Kathy who said she would take it from here. I dashed back to the house and, with the same shaving cream on my face, proceeded with my morning rituals. I remained on time for my first morning's appointment.

I have had my share of difficult deliveries, but this one remains memorable. The "shave cream delivery" is how we know it around our house.

# CHAPTER 18

*— My First Day —*

# Chapter 18

It was a hard day to be sad. All seemed to flow effortlessly. Azure blue skies with puffy white clouds signaled a glorious early summer day.

I was behind the wheel of my brand new Chevy pickup truck. I had been given a good price on it I think because the colors were beige and white and no one would buy it. While it was not perfect, it was a start for my brand new veterinary practice. I could have used a more robust suspension, four-wheel drive, and an extra seat in the back.

I had bought a "vet unit" used from the vet school. Made of white fiberglass, it consisted of doors behind which were shelves and drawers where the tools of the trade and the medicines were stored. I would soon discover a phenomenon that I called "DT's." In upstate New York the roads would suffer savage upheavals from winter frost. These miniature mountains would appear without notice and I, traveling at a speed far greater than gravity would like, would launch my truck up in the air at a sharp angle and then in a millisecond, be returned to the previous level. This sharp and abrupt directional change would, with the character of a tornado, toss everything out of the drawers and scatter vials of medicine throughout the interior of the vet unit. These bumps were soon named DT's for "drawer tossers."

The day had started with excitement. Mom was at the farm along with Kathy's parents. Everyone was dressed in their fancy clothes and we all piled into cars and drove to Cornell for my graduation. In a quiet moment, I thought I could feel Dad there along with the grandparents I had known. Both the dead and the living oozed pride that Geoff had finally made it. He had finally decided to apply himself to one goal and follow through. Mom was crying.

The next few hours were a blur. I did not want to be there in a room full of "youngsters." I was five years older than everyone because I hadn't followed the path of high school, college, and vet school. My classmates seemed so much smarter than me, though I was not the last in the class academically. Not only were they smart, but they also all seemed to be heading off to bright careers. My future was a little more tenuous.

We dressed in our gray and maroon caps and gowns, assembled in the auditorium, repeated the veterinary oath in unison, were told we were the finest class the school had had the privilege to teach, and marched off to the football stadium for the ceremony with the other schools.

We were all conferred our degrees, threw our hats into the air, inflated the plastic obstetrical sleeves and, with pudgy air filled fingers pointed skyward, waved them high to separate ourselves from the other schools graduating that day. Then we found our loved ones and in a mass of disorder, exited the stadium. Now it was back to the farm for some good eating.

My classmates returned up campus to the vet school where a tent had been erected for a reception. Maybe I should have attended, but I felt I didn't fit in. Maybe it was the age difference. Maybe it was because they were all talking about where they were relocating and that brought on sobbing and hugging. I think the real reason was I had heard they were serving cake and beer and I knew there was better food at home.

I sat on my porch with my mind drifting over the previous decade. I was in disbelief. How on earth did I get here? I had just graduated and I already had set up an ambulatory equine practice. I had named it The Finger Lakes Equine Practice and I was wearing a beeper. My ever-emotional mother came to me at this point with tears in her eyes and said, "You're wearing a pager! Now I know you are a doctor!" Geez Mom!

Not to disappoint her, the pager erupted with a high-pitched electronic alarm that at one point in later years almost killed me. It was the first of many that would have me pick up the nearest landline and call Sue or Diane at the answering service. There were no cellular phones in 1984 and these two bastions of the Ithaca Answering Service helped me build the practice over the years when Kathy was unable to answer the phone. Their calming presence helped many horse owners with their emergencies until I could be reached. Today, however, it was all business when Sue said, "Dr. Tucker, I have Janet on the line and she has a foal with a bad eye."

My first call! I had dreamed of this day. I had *prepared* with five years working with horses full time and seven years in school. The *opportunity* occurred when a rambunctious foal had injured his eye. I felt *lucky*!

Before graduation, I knew I was going to start my practice in Cornell's backyard. Many had called me crazy but local horse owners had been disappointed when they could not find adequate routine horse care from the small animal or cow vets the university would send out.

An example of this had happened when I was on the field service rotation in the spring. This was a six-week rotation where four students were assigned to a truck with a veterinary instructor and we drove to local farms to work on cows, horses, and other farm animals. Everyone knew that I was all about horses but the instructor was in charge and I had to respect his position. The rest of the students were small animal classmates required to go through this rotation in order to graduate. We visited a horse with colic that day.

This horse was very depressed while all of us took our turns doing a full exam. The five of us performed heart rate, respiratory rate, gum color, and listened to the GI tract. To me, this horse looked bad. It reminded me of the horse I had seen in California with Dr. Munson when he said to me, "This one's not going to make it."

The instructor, in a grand effort to show his authority, proclaimed that this horse needed his teeth floated then performed a very rudimentary job of it. He then told the owner he would be back in two hours to recheck the patient and we piled into the truck and left for a dairy farm.

Floating the teeth of a horse that has colic is completely senseless and was not only unnecessary, but it just added stress to the sick horse. An equivalent example would be if you, upon entering the hospital with a heart attack, had the attending emergency physician order an X-ray of your ankle. I am sure the clinician was great with cows, but like me with dogs and cats, he just was not confident of what to do.

We returned two hours later and found the horse dead. This represented one of the many reasons I stayed in Ithaca to offer horse owners an alternative in horse care. Please understand that Cornell's Veterinary School in house is the finest available. Routine horsemanship and horse husbandry however was needed at the farm level and they had difficulty providing it. I saw an opportunity.

Today with graduation a few hours earlier I had my first call. I said goodbye to the family, the first of tens of thousands of goodbyes, and went to my truck.

E-Z and I had been together for about ten years and those were pivotal years for me. A German Shepherd mix, I had adopted him from the pound and he had adopted me. We had started together at Trotter Farm and had been everywhere together including completely across the country to California and back again. But now he was in his waning days and had slowed down a lot. He was having trouble breathing at night with a soft moist cough. As a vet, I knew it was cancer and it was his last few days. But as a man, I prayed I would be able to take him on just one call together as old friends just like we always had. It had been a dream of mine since entering vet school four years ago that E-Z would make the full journey with me, from the directionless gypsies we'd started out as, to qualified caregivers that could do a lot of good for the animals we encountered. This day, I gently lifted him into the passenger seat of the truck.

I got into my side behind the wheel, started the truck, and drove onto the road. On the truck's bench seat, E-Z's head now lay on my right thigh and I gently stroked it. For all the excitement of this day, with graduation and my first official vet call, I should be happy, but the tears streamed down my face. My prayer had been answered, but I wouldn't have my friend much longer.

Silently we drove on the twisting roads to Janet's house about 40 minutes away. My mind went back to the first horse I rode, Patches in Texas, then to the horses in Mt. Rainer, Washington where I came to love the sights and sounds of a barn. My attempts to do well in school and my dropping out of various colleges should have sealed my fate but instead lead me to a calling I could have never imagined. Landing a job on a Saddlebred farm in Delaware, Ohio with no plan or knowledge; becoming sick and broke then finding a job on a Thoroughbred breeding and training farm in Bedford, NY. Looking back it all seemed like an intricate and well-designed plan that led me straight to this point and this day.

I drove past the vet school and saw the large tent set up for the reception. My class mates where in there eating cake and drinking beer. We were so different. The tires humming on the asphalt brought me back to the day I left the Thoroughbred farm and E-Z and I set out for Santa Barbara, California. I had adventures and sowed my oats, but nothing fulfilled me like working with horses.

It is an understatement that E-Z was my best friend during those years and now he and I were soon to part ways. It hurt, but there was also a peace about it too. We were both moving on to better things.

We arrived at the farm and Janet congratulated me on my graduation then put me to work. I examined the horse's eye and then thought how ironic it was that my first call was a corneal ulcer. My mind drifted back again to the Trotter Farm where a two year old had a "bad eye" and I was instructed by the trainer to "get that eye ointment" and treat her. I didn't know any different and just followed directions – which ended up costing that animal an eye.

Here it was eight years later and I was again looking at an eye and praying I would not make a mistake. Janet just smiled and said, "Right now, Geoff, I can't think of anyone else who I'd rather work on my little guy."

I was euphoric. This is what I was meant to do and it felt as comfortable as a well-worn glove. I was in the right time at the right place to have the life I'd always wanted.

E-Z and I went home together that evening. I did the talking. I did the crying. The next morning I performed the first euthanasia of my practice. EZ was finally at peace and so was I.

Lightning Source UK Ltd.
Milton Keynes UK
UKHW010454141221
395595UK00004B/1081

9 781934 606537